SCHOOL INFORMATION

SCHOOL NAME	
SCHOOL ADDRESS	
EMAIL ADDRESS	
WEBSITE	
PHONE No:	**FAX No:**

EMERGENCY CONTACT

FULLNAME	
ADDRESS	
E-MAIL ADDRESS	
PHONE No	

NOTES

_____

_____

_____

_____

_____

_____

_____

INDEX

No	INCIDENT / ACCIDENT	DATE	PAGE

No	INCIDENT / ACCIDENT	DATE	PAGE
No	INCIDENT / ACCIDENT	DATE	PAGE

No	INCIDENT / ACCIDENT	DATE	PAGE

INDEX

INDEX

No	INCIDENT / ACCIDENT	DATE	PAGE

CHILDMINDING ACCIDENT/ INCIDENT REPORT

INCIDENT NO:	INCIDENT DATE:		INCIDENT TIME:
LOCATION:	REPORTED TIME:		REPORTED DATE:
PERSON INJURED / INVOLVED	O STUDENT O ACADEMIC STAFF		O NON-ACADEMIC STAFF
	O VISITOR O OTHER :		
FULLNAME:		CLASS:	
ADDRESS:			
NATURE & EXTENT OF INJURIES	O GRAZE O BUMP O CUT O FALL O NOSEBLEED		
	O SCRATCHES O OTHER:		

DETAILS OF INCIDENT / ACCIDENT

WHAT ACTION WAS TAKEN ?	O FIRST AID O AMBULLANCE CALLED O HOSPITAL O POLICE
	O OTHER:

WITNESS (ES)	ACTION (S) WHICH COULD HAVE PREVENTED THE INCIDENT
1.	
2.	
3.	

EMERGENCY CONTACT (PARENT / GUARDIAN INFORMATION)

FULLNAME:		
E-MAIL ADDRESS:		PHONE No:
OUTCOME	O PARENT SPOKEN TO O VOICEMAIL	O NO ANSWER
CONTACT MADE BY:		TIME:
INCIDENT HANDLED BY:		
TREATMENT GIVEN BY:		
FORM COMPLETED BY:		
POSITION:		DATE:
APPROVED BY:		
POSITION:		DATE:

CHILDMINDING ACCIDENT/ INCIDENT REPORT

INCIDENT NO:	INCIDENT DATE:	INCIDENT TIME:
LOCATION:	REPORTED TIME:	REPORTED DATE:

PERSON INJURED / INVOLVED	○ STUDENT ○ ACADEMIC STAFF ○ NON-ACADEMIC STAFF ○ VISITOR ○ OTHER :

FULLNAME:	CLASS:

ADDRESS:

NATURE & EXTENT OF INJURIES	○ GRAZE ○ BUMP ○ CUT ○ FALL ○ NOSEBLEED ○ SCRATCHES ○ OTHER:

DETAILS OF INCIDENT / ACCIDENT

WHAT ACTION WAS TAKEN ?	○ FIRST AID ○ AMBULLANCE CALLED ○ HOSPITAL ○ POLICE ○ OTHER:

WITNESS (ES)	ACTION (S) WHICH COULD HAVE PREVENTED THE INCIDENT
1.	
2.	
3.	

EMERGENCY CONTACT (PARENT / GUARDIAN INFORMATION)

FULLNAME:	
E-MAIL ADDRESS:	PHONE No:
OUTCOME	○ PARENT SPOKEN TO ○ VOICEMAIL ○ NO ANSWER
CONTACT MADE BY:	TIME:
INCIDENT HANDLED BY:	
TREATMENT GIVEN BY:	
FORM COMPLETED BY:	
POSITION:	DATE:
APPROVED BY:	
POSITION:	DATE:

CHILDMINDING ACCIDENT/ INCIDENT REPORT

INCIDENT NO:	INCIDENT DATE:	INCIDENT TIME:
LOCATION:	REPORTED TIME:	REPORTED DATE:

PERSON INJURED / INVOLVED	○ STUDENT ○ ACADEMIC STAFF ○ NON-ACADEMIC STAFF ○ VISITOR ○ OTHER :

FULLNAME:		CLASS:

ADDRESS:		

NATURE & EXTENT OF INJURIES	○ GRAZE ○ BUMP ○ CUT ○ FALL ○ NOSEBLEED ○ SCRATCHES ○ OTHER:

DETAILS OF INCIDENT / ACCIDENT

WHAT ACTION WAS TAKEN ?	○ FIRST AID ○ AMBULLANCE CALLED ○ HOSPITAL ○ POLICE ○ OTHER:

WITNESS (ES)	ACTION (S) WHICH COULD HAVE PREVENTED THE INCIDENT
1.	
2.	
3.	

EMERGENCY CONTACT (PARENT / GUARDIAN INFORMATION)

FULLNAME:		
E-MAIL ADDRESS:		PHONE No:
OUTCOME	○ PARENT SPOKEN TO ○ VOICEMAIL	○ NO ANSWER
CONTACT MADE BY:		TIME:
INCIDENT HANDLED BY:		
TREATMENT GIVEN BY:		
FORM COMPLETED BY:		
POSITION:		DATE:
APPROVED BY:		
POSITION:		DATE:

CHILDMINDING ACCIDENT/ INCIDENT REPORT

INCIDENT NO:	INCIDENT DATE:	INCIDENT TIME:
LOCATION:	REPORTED TIME:	REPORTED DATE:

PERSON INJURED / INVOLVED	O STUDENT O ACADEMIC STAFF O NON-ACADEMIC STAFF O VISITOR O OTHER :	

FULLNAME:		CLASS:

ADDRESS:		

NATURE & EXTENT OF INJURIES	O GRAZE O BUMP O CUT O FALL O NOSEBLEED O SCRATCHES O OTHER:	

DETAILS OF INCIDENT / ACCIDENT

WHAT ACTION WAS TAKEN ?	O FIRST AID O AMBULLANCE CALLED O HOSPITAL O POLICE O OTHER:

WITNESS (ES)	ACTION (S) WHICH COULD HAVE PREVENTED THE INCIDENT
1.	
2.	
3.	

EMERGENCY CONTACT (PARENT / GUARDIAN INFORMATION)

FULLNAME:		
E-MAIL ADDRESS:		PHONE No:
OUTCOME	O PARENT SPOKEN TO O VOICEMAIL O NO ANSWER	
CONTACT MADE BY:		TIME:
INCIDENT HANDLED BY:		
TREATMENT GIVEN BY:		
FORM COMPLETED BY:		
POSITION:		DATE:
APPROVED BY:		
POSITION:		DATE:

CHILDMINDING ACCIDENT/ INCIDENT REPORT

INCIDENT NO:	INCIDENT DATE:	INCIDENT TIME:
LOCATION:	REPORTED TIME:	REPORTED DATE:

PERSON INJURED / INVOLVED	○ STUDENT ○ ACADEMIC STAFF ○ NON-ACADEMIC STAFF ○ VISITOR ○ OTHER :		

FULLNAME:	CLASS:

ADDRESS:	

NATURE & EXTENT OF INJURIES	○ GRAZE ○ BUMP ○ CUT ○ FALL ○ NOSEBLEED ○ SCRATCHES ○ OTHER:

DETAILS OF INCIDENT / ACCIDENT

WHAT ACTION WAS TAKEN ?	○ FIRST AID ○ AMBULLANCE CALLED ○ HOSPITAL ○ POLICE ○ OTHER:

WITNESS (ES)	ACTION (S) WHICH COULD HAVE PREVENTED THE INCIDENT
1.	
2.	
3.	

EMERGENCY CONTACT (PARENT / GUARDIAN INFORMATION)

FULLNAME:		
E-MAIL ADDRESS:	PHONE No:	
OUTCOME	○ PARENT SPOKEN TO ○ VOICEMAIL ○ NO ANSWER	
CONTACT MADE BY:	TIME:	
INCIDENT HANDLED BY:		
TREATMENT GIVEN BY:		
FORM COMPLETED BY:		
POSITION:	DATE:	
APPROVED BY:		
POSITION:	DATE:	

CHILDMINDING ACCIDENT/ INCIDENT REPORT

INCIDENT NO:	INCIDENT DATE:	INCIDENT TIME:
LOCATION:	REPORTED TIME:	REPORTED DATE:

PERSON INJURED / INVOLVED	O STUDENT O ACADEMIC STAFF O NON-ACADEMIC STAFF O VISITOR O OTHER :	
FULLNAME:		CLASS:
ADDRESS:		
NATURE & EXTENT OF INJURIES	O GRAZE O BUMP O CUT O FALL O NOSEBLEED O SCRATCHES O OTHER:	

DETAILS OF INCIDENT / ACCIDENT

WHAT ACTION WAS TAKEN ?	O FIRST AID O AMBULLANCE CALLED O HOSPITAL O POLICE O OTHER:

WITNESS (ES)	ACTION (S) WHICH COULD HAVE PREVENTED THE INCIDENT
1.	
2.	
3.	

EMERGENCY CONTACT (PARENT / GUARDIAN INFORMATION)

FULLNAME:		
E-MAIL ADDRESS:		PHONE No:
OUTCOME	O PARENT SPOKEN TO O VOICEMAIL O NO ANSWER	
CONTACT MADE BY:		TIME:
INCIDENT HANDLED BY:		
TREATMENT GIVEN BY:		
FORM COMPLETED BY:		
POSITION:		DATE:
APPROVED BY:		
POSITION:		DATE:

CHILDMINDING ACCIDENT/ INCIDENT REPORT

INCIDENT NO:	INCIDENT DATE:	INCIDENT TIME:
LOCATION:	REPORTED TIME:	REPORTED DATE:

PERSON INJURED / INVOLVED	○ STUDENT ○ ACADEMIC STAFF ○ NON-ACADEMIC STAFF ○ VISITOR ○ OTHER :	

FULLNAME:		CLASS:

ADDRESS:		

NATURE & EXTENT OF INJURIES	○ GRAZE ○ BUMP ○ CUT ○ FALL ○ NOSEBLEED ○ SCRATCHES ○ OTHER:	

DETAILS OF INCIDENT / ACCIDENT

WHAT ACTION WAS TAKEN ?	○ FIRST AID ○ AMBULLANCE CALLED ○ HOSPITAL ○ POLICE ○ OTHER:	

WITNESS (ES)	ACTION (S) WHICH COULD HAVE PREVENTED THE INCIDENT
1.	
2.	
3.	

EMERGENCY CONTACT (PARENT / GUARDIAN INFORMATION)

FULLNAME:		
E-MAIL ADDRESS:		PHONE No:
OUTCOME	○ PARENT SPOKEN TO ○ VOICEMAIL ○ NO ANSWER	
CONTACT MADE BY:		TIME:
INCIDENT HANDLED BY:		
TREATMENT GIVEN BY:		
FORM COMPLETED BY:		
POSITION:		DATE:
APPROVED BY:		
POSITION:		DATE:

CHILDMINDING ACCIDENT/ INCIDENT REPORT

INCIDENT NO:	INCIDENT DATE:	INCIDENT TIME:
LOCATION:	REPORTED TIME:	REPORTED DATE:

PERSON INJURED / INVOLVED	O STUDENT O ACADEMIC STAFF O NON-ACADEMIC STAFF O VISITOR O OTHER :

FULLNAME:	CLASS:

ADDRESS:	

NATURE & EXTENT OF INJURIES	O GRAZE O BUMP O CUT O FALL O NOSEBLEED O SCRATCHES O OTHER:

DETAILS OF INCIDENT / ACCIDENT

WHAT ACTION WAS TAKEN ?	O FIRST AID O AMBULLANCE CALLED O HOSPITAL O POLICE O OTHER:

WITNESS (ES)	ACTION (S) WHICH COULD HAVE PREVENTED THE INCIDENT
1.	
2.	
3.	

EMERGENCY CONTACT (PARENT / GUARDIAN INFORMATION)

FULLNAME:	
E-MAIL ADDRESS:	PHONE No:
OUTCOME	O PARENT SPOKEN TO O VOICEMAIL O NO ANSWER
CONTACT MADE BY:	TIME:
INCIDENT HANDLED BY:	
TREATMENT GIVEN BY:	
FORM COMPLETED BY:	
POSITION:	DATE:
APPROVED BY:	
POSITION:	DATE:

CHILDMINDING ACCIDENT/ INCIDENT REPORT

INCIDENT NO:	INCIDENT DATE:	INCIDENT TIME:
LOCATION:	REPORTED TIME:	REPORTED DATE:

PERSON INJURED / INVOLVED	○ STUDENT ○ ACADEMIC STAFF ○ NON-ACADEMIC STAFF ○ VISITOR ○ OTHER :

FULLNAME:	CLASS:

ADDRESS:	

NATURE & EXTENT OF INJURIES	○ GRAZE ○ BUMP ○ CUT ○ FALL ○ NOSEBLEED ○ SCRATCHES ○ OTHER:

DETAILS OF INCIDENT / ACCIDENT

WHAT ACTION WAS TAKEN ?	○ FIRST AID ○ AMBULLANCE CALLED ○ HOSPITAL ○ POLICE ○ OTHER:

WITNESS (ES)	ACTION (S) WHICH COULD HAVE PREVENTED THE INCIDENT
1.	
2.	
3.	

EMERGENCY CONTACT (PARENT / GUARDIAN INFORMATION)

FULLNAME:		
E-MAIL ADDRESS:	PHONE No:	
OUTCOME	○ PARENT SPOKEN TO ○ VOICEMAIL ○ NO ANSWER	
CONTACT MADE BY:	TIME:	
INCIDENT HANDLED BY:		
TREATMENT GIVEN BY:		
FORM COMPLETED BY:		
POSITION:	DATE:	
APPROVED BY:		
POSITION:	DATE:	

CHILDMINDING ACCIDENT/ INCIDENT REPORT

INCIDENT NO:	INCIDENT DATE:	INCIDENT TIME:
LOCATION:	REPORTED TIME:	REPORTED DATE:

| PERSON INJURED / INVOLVED | ○ STUDENT ○ ACADEMIC STAFF ○ NON-ACADEMIC STAFF ○ VISITOR ○ OTHER : | | |

FULLNAME:		CLASS:

ADDRESS:

NATURE & EXTENT OF INJURIES	○ GRAZE ○ BUMP ○ CUT ○ FALL ○ NOSEBLEED ○ SCRATCHES ○ OTHER:

DETAILS OF INCIDENT / ACCIDENT

WHAT ACTION WAS TAKEN ?	○ FIRST AID ○ AMBULLANCE CALLED ○ HOSPITAL ○ POLICE ○ OTHER:

WITNESS (ES)	ACTION (S) WHICH COULD HAVE PREVENTED THE INCIDENT
1.	
2.	
3.	

EMERGENCY CONTACT (PARENT / GUARDIAN INFORMATION)

FULLNAME:		
E-MAIL ADDRESS:		PHONE No:
OUTCOME	○ PARENT SPOKEN TO ○ VOICEMAIL	○ NO ANSWER
CONTACT MADE BY:		TIME:
INCIDENT HANDLED BY:		
TREATMENT GIVEN BY:		
FORM COMPLETED BY:		
POSITION:		DATE:
APPROVED BY:		
POSITION:		DATE:

CHILDMINDING ACCIDENT/ INCIDENT REPORT

INCIDENT NO:	INCIDENT DATE:	INCIDENT TIME:
LOCATION:	REPORTED TIME:	REPORTED DATE:

PERSON INJURED / INVOLVED	O STUDENT O ACADEMIC STAFF O NON-ACADEMIC STAFF O VISITOR O OTHER :		

FULLNAME:		CLASS:

ADDRESS:		

NATURE & EXTENT OF INJURIES	O GRAZE O BUMP O CUT O FALL O NOSEBLEED O SCRATCHES O OTHER:

DETAILS OF INCIDENT / ACCIDENT

WHAT ACTION WAS TAKEN ?	O FIRST AID O AMBULLANCE CALLED O HOSPITAL O POLICE O OTHER:

WITNESS (ES)	ACTION (S) WHICH COULD HAVE PREVENTED THE INCIDENT
1.	
2.	
3.	

EMERGENCY CONTACT (PARENT / GUARDIAN INFORMATION)

FULLNAME:		
E-MAIL ADDRESS:		PHONE No:
OUTCOME	O PARENT SPOKEN TO O VOICEMAIL O NO ANSWER	
CONTACT MADE BY:		TIME:
INCIDENT HANDLED BY:		
TREATMENT GIVEN BY:		
FORM COMPLETED BY:		
POSITION:		DATE:
APPROVED BY:		
POSITION:		DATE:

CHILDMINDING ACCIDENT/ INCIDENT REPORT

INCIDENT NO:	INCIDENT DATE:	INCIDENT TIME:
LOCATION:	REPORTED TIME:	REPORTED DATE:

PERSON INJURED / INVOLVED	O STUDENT O ACADEMIC STAFF O NON-ACADEMIC STAFF O VISITOR O OTHER :	

FULLNAME:		CLASS:

ADDRESS:

NATURE & EXTENT OF INJURIES	O GRAZE O BUMP O CUT O FALL O NOSEBLEED O SCRATCHES O OTHER:

DETAILS OF INCIDENT / ACCIDENT

WHAT ACTION WAS TAKEN ?	O FIRST AID O AMBULLANCE CALLED O HOSPITAL O POLICE O OTHER:

WITNESS (ES)	ACTION (S) WHICH COULD HAVE PREVENTED THE INCIDENT
1.	
2.	
3.	

EMERGENCY CONTACT (PARENT / GUARDIAN INFORMATION)

FULLNAME:		
E-MAIL ADDRESS:		PHONE No:
OUTCOME	O PARENT SPOKEN TO O VOICEMAIL	O NO ANSWER
CONTACT MADE BY:		TIME:
INCIDENT HANDLED BY:		
TREATMENT GIVEN BY:		
FORM COMPLETED BY:		
POSITION:		DATE:
APPROVED BY:		
POSITION:		DATE:

CHILDMINDING ACCIDENT/ INCIDENT REPORT

INCIDENT NO:	INCIDENT DATE:	INCIDENT TIME:
LOCATION:	REPORTED TIME:	REPORTED DATE:

PERSON INJURED / INVOLVED	O STUDENT O ACADEMIC STAFF O NON-ACADEMIC STAFF O VISITOR O OTHER :

FULLNAME:	CLASS:

ADDRESS:	

NATURE & EXTENT OF INJURIES	O GRAZE O BUMP O CUT O FALL O NOSEBLEED O SCRATCHES O OTHER:

DETAILS OF INCIDENT / ACCIDENT

WHAT ACTION WAS TAKEN ?	O FIRST AID O AMBULLANCE CALLED O HOSPITAL O POLICE O OTHER:

WITNESS (ES)	ACTION (S) WHICH COULD HAVE PREVENTED THE INCIDENT
1.	
2.	
3.	

EMERGENCY CONTACT (PARENT / GUARDIAN INFORMATION)

FULLNAME:		
E-MAIL ADDRESS:		PHONE No:
OUTCOME	O PARENT SPOKEN TO O VOICEMAIL O NO ANSWER	
CONTACT MADE BY:		TIME:
INCIDENT HANDLED BY:		
TREATMENT GIVEN BY:		
FORM COMPLETED BY:		
POSITION:		DATE:
APPROVED BY:		
POSITION:		DATE:

CHILDMINDING ACCIDENT/ INCIDENT REPORT

INCIDENT NO:	INCIDENT DATE:	INCIDENT TIME:
LOCATION:	REPORTED TIME:	REPORTED DATE:
PERSON INJURED / INVOLVED	○ STUDENT ○ ACADEMIC STAFF ○ NON-ACADEMIC STAFF ○ VISITOR ○ OTHER :	
FULLNAME:		CLASS:
ADDRESS:		
NATURE & EXTENT OF INJURIES	○ GRAZE ○ BUMP ○ CUT ○ FALL ○ NOSEBLEED ○ SCRATCHES ○ OTHER:	

DETAILS OF INCIDENT / ACCIDENT

WHAT ACTION WAS TAKEN ?	○ FIRST AID ○ AMBULLANCE CALLED ○ HOSPITAL ○ POLICE ○ OTHER:	

WITNESS (ES)	ACTION (S) WHICH COULD HAVE PREVENTED THE INCIDENT
1.	
2.	
3.	

EMERGENCY CONTACT (PARENT / GUARDIAN INFORMATION)

FULLNAME:		
E-MAIL ADDRESS:		PHONE No:
OUTCOME	○ PARENT SPOKEN TO ○ VOICEMAIL	○ NO ANSWER
CONTACT MADE BY:		TIME:
INCIDENT HANDLED BY:		
TREATMENT GIVEN BY:		
FORM COMPLETED BY:		
POSITION:		DATE:
APPROVED BY:		
POSITION:		DATE:

CHILDMINDING ACCIDENT/ INCIDENT REPORT

INCIDENT NO:	INCIDENT DATE:	INCIDENT TIME:
LOCATION:	REPORTED TIME:	REPORTED DATE:

| PERSON INJURED / INVOLVED | ○ STUDENT ○ ACADEMIC STAFF ○ NON-ACADEMIC STAFF
 ○ VISITOR ○ OTHER : | |

FULLNAME:		CLASS:

ADDRESS:		

NATURE & EXTENT OF INJURIES	○ GRAZE ○ BUMP ○ CUT ○ FALL ○ NOSEBLEED ○ SCRATCHES ○ OTHER:

DETAILS OF INCIDENT / ACCIDENT

WHAT ACTION WAS TAKEN ?	○ FIRST AID ○ AMBULLANCE CALLED ○ HOSPITAL ○ POLICE ○ OTHER:

WITNESS (ES)	ACTION (S) WHICH COULD HAVE PREVENTED THE INCIDENT
1.	
2.	
3.	

EMERGENCY CONTACT (PARENT / GUARDIAN INFORMATION)

FULLNAME:		
E-MAIL ADDRESS:		PHONE No:
OUTCOME	○ PARENT SPOKEN TO ○ VOICEMAIL ○ NO ANSWER	
CONTACT MADE BY:		TIME:
INCIDENT HANDLED BY:		
TREATMENT GIVEN BY:		
FORM COMPLETED BY:		
POSITION:		DATE:
APPROVED BY:		
POSITION:		DATE:

CHILDMINDING ACCIDENT/ INCIDENT REPORT

INCIDENT NO:	**INCIDENT DATE:**	**INCIDENT TIME:**
LOCATION:	**REPORTED TIME:**	**REPORTED DATE:**

PERSON INJURED / INVOLVED	O STUDENT	O ACADEMIC STAFF	O NON-ACADEMIC STAFF
	O VISITOR	O OTHER :	

FULLNAME:		**CLASS:**

ADDRESS:

NATURE & EXTENT OF INJURIES	O GRAZE	O BUMP	O CUT	O FALL	O NOSEBLEED
	O SCRATCHES	O OTHER:			

DETAILS OF INCIDENT / ACCIDENT

WHAT ACTION WAS TAKEN ?	O FIRST AID	O AMBULLANCE CALLED	O HOSPITAL	O POLICE
	O OTHER:			

WITNESS (ES)	ACTION (S) WHICH COULD HAVE PREVENTED THE INCIDENT
1.	
2.	
3.	

EMERGENCY CONTACT (PARENT / GUARDIAN INFORMATION)

FULLNAME:		
E-MAIL ADDRESS:		**PHONE No:**

OUTCOME	O PARENT SPOKEN TO	O VOICEMAIL	O NO ANSWER

CONTACT MADE BY:		**TIME:**
INCIDENT HANDLED BY:		
TREATMENT GIVEN BY:		
FORM COMPLETED BY:		
POSITION:		**DATE:**
APPROVED BY:		
POSITION:		**DATE:**

CHILDMINDING ACCIDENT/ INCIDENT REPORT

INCIDENT NO:	INCIDENT DATE:	INCIDENT TIME:
LOCATION:	REPORTED TIME:	REPORTED DATE:

| PERSON INJURED / INVOLVED | O STUDENT   O ACADEMIC STAFF   O NON-ACADEMIC STAFF
 O VISITOR   O OTHER : |||

FULLNAME:		CLASS:
ADDRESS:		

| NATURE & EXTENT OF INJURIES | O GRAZE   O BUMP   O CUT   O FALL   O NOSEBLEED
 O SCRATCHES   O OTHER: |

DETAILS OF INCIDENT / ACCIDENT

WHAT ACTION WAS TAKEN ?	O FIRST AID O AMBULLANCE CALLED O HOSPITAL O POLICE O OTHER:

WITNESS (ES)	ACTION (S) WHICH COULD HAVE PREVENTED THE INCIDENT
1.	
2.	
3.	

EMERGENCY CONTACT (PARENT / GUARDIAN INFORMATION)

FULLNAME:		
E-MAIL ADDRESS:		PHONE No:
OUTCOME	O PARENT SPOKEN TO O VOICEMAIL O NO ANSWER	
CONTACT MADE BY:		TIME:
INCIDENT HANDLED BY:		
TREATMENT GIVEN BY:		
FORM COMPLETED BY:		
POSITION:		DATE:
APPROVED BY:		
POSITION:		DATE:

CHILDMINDING ACCIDENT/ INCIDENT REPORT

INCIDENT NO:	INCIDENT DATE:		INCIDENT TIME:	
LOCATION:	REPORTED TIME:		REPORTED DATE:	
PERSON INJURED / INVOLVED	O STUDENT O ACADEMIC STAFF		O NON-ACADEMIC STAFF	
	O VISITOR O OTHER :			
FULLNAME:			CLASS:	
ADDRESS:				
NATURE & EXTENT OF INJURIES	O GRAZE O BUMP O CUT O FALL O NOSEBLEED			
	O SCRATCHES O OTHER:			

DETAILS OF INCIDENT / ACCIDENT

WHAT ACTION WAS TAKEN ?	O FIRST AID O AMBULLANCE CALLED O HOSPITAL O POLICE
	O OTHER:

WITNESS (ES)	ACTION (S) WHICH COULD HAVE PREVENTED THE INCIDENT
1.	
2.	
3.	

EMERGENCY CONTACT (PARENT / GUARDIAN INFORMATION)

FULLNAME:			
E-MAIL ADDRESS:		PHONE No:	
OUTCOME	O PARENT SPOKEN TO	O VOICEMAIL	O NO ANSWER
CONTACT MADE BY:		TIME:	
INCIDENT HANDLED BY:			
TREATMENT GIVEN BY:			
FORM COMPLETED BY:			
POSITION:		DATE:	
APPROVED BY:			
POSITION:		DATE:	

CHILDMINDING ACCIDENT/ INCIDENT REPORT

INCIDENT NO:	INCIDENT DATE:	INCIDENT TIME:
LOCATION:	REPORTED TIME:	REPORTED DATE:

| PERSON INJURED / INVOLVED | O STUDENT   O ACADEMIC STAFF   O NON-ACADEMIC STAFF
 O VISITOR   O OTHER : |||

FULLNAME:		CLASS:
ADDRESS:			

| NATURE & EXTENT OF INJURIES | O GRAZE   O BUMP   O CUT   O FALL   O NOSEBLEED
 O SCRATCHES   O OTHER: |

DETAILS OF INCIDENT / ACCIDENT

| WHAT ACTION WAS TAKEN ? | O FIRST AID   O AMBULLANCE CALLED   O HOSPITAL   O POLICE
 O OTHER: |

WITNESS (ES)	ACTION (S) WHICH COULD HAVE PREVENTED THE INCIDENT
1.	
2.	
3.	

EMERGENCY CONTACT (PARENT / GUARDIAN INFORMATION)

FULLNAME:		
E-MAIL ADDRESS:		PHONE No:
OUTCOME	O PARENT SPOKEN TO O VOICEMAIL O NO ANSWER	
CONTACT MADE BY:		TIME:
INCIDENT HANDLED BY:		
TREATMENT GIVEN BY:		
FORM COMPLETED BY:		
POSITION:		DATE:
APPROVED BY:		
POSITION:		DATE:

CHILDMINDING ACCIDENT/ INCIDENT REPORT

INCIDENT NO:	INCIDENT DATE:	INCIDENT TIME:
LOCATION:	REPORTED TIME:	REPORTED DATE:

PERSON INJURED / INVOLVED	○ STUDENT ○ ACADEMIC STAFF ○ NON-ACADEMIC STAFF ○ VISITOR ○ OTHER :	

FULLNAME:		CLASS:

ADDRESS:		

NATURE & EXTENT OF INJURIES	○ GRAZE ○ BUMP ○ CUT ○ FALL ○ NOSEBLEED ○ SCRATCHES ○ OTHER:

DETAILS OF INCIDENT / ACCIDENT

WHAT ACTION WAS TAKEN ?	○ FIRST AID ○ AMBULLANCE CALLED ○ HOSPITAL ○ POLICE ○ OTHER:

WITNESS (ES)	ACTION (S) WHICH COULD HAVE PREVENTED THE INCIDENT
1.	
2.	
3.	

EMERGENCY CONTACT (PARENT / GUARDIAN INFORMATION)

FULLNAME:		
E-MAIL ADDRESS:		PHONE No:
OUTCOME	○ PARENT SPOKEN TO ○ VOICEMAIL ○ NO ANSWER	
CONTACT MADE BY:		TIME:
INCIDENT HANDLED BY:		
TREATMENT GIVEN BY:		
FORM COMPLETED BY:		
POSITION:		DATE:
APPROVED BY:		
POSITION:		DATE:

CHILDMINDING ACCIDENT/ INCIDENT REPORT

INCIDENT NO:	INCIDENT DATE:	INCIDENT TIME:
LOCATION:	REPORTED TIME:	REPORTED DATE:

PERSON INJURED / INVOLVED	O STUDENT O ACADEMIC STAFF O NON-ACADEMIC STAFF O VISITOR O OTHER :

FULLNAME:	CLASS:

ADDRESS:	

NATURE & EXTENT OF INJURIES	O GRAZE O BUMP O CUT O FALL O NOSEBLEED O SCRATCHES O OTHER:

DETAILS OF INCIDENT / ACCIDENT

WHAT ACTION WAS TAKEN ?	O FIRST AID O AMBULLANCE CALLED O HOSPITAL O POLICE O OTHER:

WITNESS (ES)	ACTION (S) WHICH COULD HAVE PREVENTED THE INCIDENT
1.	
2.	
3.	

EMERGENCY CONTACT (PARENT / GUARDIAN INFORMATION)

FULLNAME:	
E-MAIL ADDRESS:	PHONE No:
OUTCOME	O PARENT SPOKEN TO O VOICEMAIL O NO ANSWER
CONTACT MADE BY:	TIME:
INCIDENT HANDLED BY:	
TREATMENT GIVEN BY:	
FORM COMPLETED BY:	
POSITION:	DATE:
APPROVED BY:	
POSITION:	DATE:

CHILDMINDING ACCIDENT/ INCIDENT REPORT

INCIDENT NO:	INCIDENT DATE:		INCIDENT TIME:
LOCATION:	REPORTED TIME:		REPORTED DATE:
PERSON INJURED / INVOLVED	O STUDENT O ACADEMIC STAFF O NON-ACADEMIC STAFF O VISITOR O OTHER :		
FULLNAME:		CLASS:	
ADDRESS:			
NATURE & EXTENT OF INJURIES	O GRAZE O BUMP O CUT O FALL O NOSEBLEED O SCRATCHES O OTHER:		

DETAILS OF INCIDENT / ACCIDENT

WHAT ACTION WAS TAKEN ?	O FIRST AID O AMBULLANCE CALLED O HOSPITAL O POLICE O OTHER:

WITNESS (ES)	ACTION (S) WHICH COULD HAVE PREVENTED THE INCIDENT
1.	
2.	
3.	

EMERGENCY CONTACT (PARENT / GUARDIAN INFORMATION)

FULLNAME:		
E-MAIL ADDRESS:		PHONE No:
OUTCOME	O PARENT SPOKEN TO O VOICEMAIL O NO ANSWER	
CONTACT MADE BY:		TIME:
INCIDENT HANDLED BY:		
TREATMENT GIVEN BY:		
FORM COMPLETED BY:		
POSITION:		DATE:
APPROVED BY:		
POSITION:		DATE:

CHILDMINDING ACCIDENT/ INCIDENT REPORT

INCIDENT NO:	INCIDENT DATE:	INCIDENT TIME:
LOCATION:	REPORTED TIME:	REPORTED DATE:

PERSON INJURED / INVOLVED	○ STUDENT ○ ACADEMIC STAFF ○ NON-ACADEMIC STAFF ○ VISITOR ○ OTHER :

FULLNAME:		CLASS:
ADDRESS:		

NATURE & EXTENT OF INJURIES	○ GRAZE ○ BUMP ○ CUT ○ FALL ○ NOSEBLEED ○ SCRATCHES ○ OTHER:

DETAILS OF INCIDENT / ACCIDENT

WHAT ACTION WAS TAKEN ?	○ FIRST AID ○ AMBULLANCE CALLED ○ HOSPITAL ○ POLICE ○ OTHER:

WITNESS (ES)	ACTION (S) WHICH COULD HAVE PREVENTED THE INCIDENT
1.	
2.	
3.	

EMERGENCY CONTACT (PARENT / GUARDIAN INFORMATION)

FULLNAME:		
E-MAIL ADDRESS:		PHONE No:
OUTCOME	○ PARENT SPOKEN TO ○ VOICEMAIL	○ NO ANSWER
CONTACT MADE BY:		TIME:
INCIDENT HANDLED BY:		
TREATMENT GIVEN BY:		
FORM COMPLETED BY:		
POSITION:		DATE:
APPROVED BY:		
POSITION:		DATE:

CHILDMINDING ACCIDENT/ INCIDENT REPORT

INCIDENT NO:	INCIDENT DATE:	INCIDENT TIME:
LOCATION:	REPORTED TIME:	REPORTED DATE:

PERSON INJURED / INVOLVED	O STUDENT O ACADEMIC STAFF O NON-ACADEMIC STAFF O VISITOR O OTHER :

FULLNAME:	CLASS:

ADDRESS:	

NATURE & EXTENT OF INJURIES	O GRAZE O BUMP O CUT O FALL O NOSEBLEED O SCRATCHES O OTHER:

DETAILS OF INCIDENT / ACCIDENT

WHAT ACTION WAS TAKEN ?	O FIRST AID O AMBULLANCE CALLED O HOSPITAL O POLICE O OTHER:

WITNESS (ES)	ACTION (S) WHICH COULD HAVE PREVENTED THE INCIDENT
1.	
2.	
3.	

EMERGENCY CONTACT (PARENT / GUARDIAN INFORMATION)

FULLNAME:		
E-MAIL ADDRESS:	PHONE No:	
OUTCOME	O PARENT SPOKEN TO O VOICEMAIL O NO ANSWER	
CONTACT MADE BY:	TIME:	
INCIDENT HANDLED BY:		
TREATMENT GIVEN BY:		
FORM COMPLETED BY:		
POSITION:	DATE:	
APPROVED BY:		
POSITION:	DATE:	

CHILDMINDING ACCIDENT/ INCIDENT REPORT

INCIDENT NO:	INCIDENT DATE:	INCIDENT TIME:
LOCATION:	REPORTED TIME:	REPORTED DATE:

PERSON INJURED / INVOLVED	○ STUDENT ○ ACADEMIC STAFF ○ NON-ACADEMIC STAFF ○ VISITOR ○ OTHER :

FULLNAME:		CLASS:

ADDRESS:		

NATURE & EXTENT OF INJURIES	○ GRAZE ○ BUMP ○ CUT ○ FALL ○ NOSEBLEED ○ SCRATCHES ○ OTHER:

DETAILS OF INCIDENT / ACCIDENT

WHAT ACTION WAS TAKEN ?	○ FIRST AID ○ AMBULLANCE CALLED ○ HOSPITAL ○ POLICE ○ OTHER:

WITNESS (ES)	ACTION (S) WHICH COULD HAVE PREVENTED THE INCIDENT
1.	
2.	
3.	

EMERGENCY CONTACT (PARENT / GUARDIAN INFORMATION)

FULLNAME:		
E-MAIL ADDRESS:		PHONE No:
OUTCOME	○ PARENT SPOKEN TO ○ VOICEMAIL ○ NO ANSWER	
CONTACT MADE BY:		TIME:
INCIDENT HANDLED BY:		
TREATMENT GIVEN BY:		
FORM COMPLETED BY:		
POSITION:		DATE:
APPROVED BY:		
POSITION:		DATE:

CHILDMINDING ACCIDENT/ INCIDENT REPORT

INCIDENT NO:	INCIDENT DATE:	INCIDENT TIME:
LOCATION:	REPORTED TIME:	REPORTED DATE:

PERSON INJURED / INVOLVED	○ STUDENT ○ ACADEMIC STAFF ○ NON-ACADEMIC STAFF ○ VISITOR ○ OTHER :

FULLNAME:	CLASS:

ADDRESS:

NATURE & EXTENT OF INJURIES	○ GRAZE ○ BUMP ○ CUT ○ FALL ○ NOSEBLEED ○ SCRATCHES ○ OTHER:

DETAILS OF INCIDENT / ACCIDENT

WHAT ACTION WAS TAKEN ?	○ FIRST AID ○ AMBULLANCE CALLED ○ HOSPITAL ○ POLICE ○ OTHER:

WITNESS (ES)	ACTION (S) WHICH COULD HAVE PREVENTED THE INCIDENT
1.	
2.	
3.	

EMERGENCY CONTACT (PARENT / GUARDIAN INFORMATION)

FULLNAME:	
E-MAIL ADDRESS:	PHONE No:
OUTCOME	○ PARENT SPOKEN TO ○ VOICEMAIL ○ NO ANSWER
CONTACT MADE BY:	TIME:
INCIDENT HANDLED BY:	
TREATMENT GIVEN BY:	
FORM COMPLETED BY:	
POSITION:	DATE:
APPROVED BY:	
POSITION:	DATE:

CHILDMINDING ACCIDENT/ INCIDENT REPORT

INCIDENT NO:	INCIDENT DATE:		INCIDENT TIME:
LOCATION:	REPORTED TIME:		REPORTED DATE:
PERSON INJURED / INVOLVED	O STUDENT O ACADEMIC STAFF O NON-ACADEMIC STAFF O VISITOR O OTHER :		
FULLNAME:		CLASS:	
ADDRESS:			
NATURE & EXTENT OF INJURIES	O GRAZE O BUMP O CUT O FALL O NOSEBLEED O SCRATCHES O OTHER:		

DETAILS OF INCIDENT / ACCIDENT

WHAT ACTION WAS TAKEN ?	O FIRST AID O AMBULLANCE CALLED O HOSPITAL O POLICE O OTHER:

WITNESS (ES)	ACTION (S) WHICH COULD HAVE PREVENTED THE INCIDENT
1.	
2.	
3.	

EMERGENCY CONTACT (PARENT / GUARDIAN INFORMATION)

FULLNAME:			
E-MAIL ADDRESS:		PHONE No:	
OUTCOME	O PARENT SPOKEN TO O VOICEMAIL O NO ANSWER		
CONTACT MADE BY:		TIME:	
INCIDENT HANDLED BY:			
TREATMENT GIVEN BY:			
FORM COMPLETED BY:			
POSITION:		DATE:	
APPROVED BY:			
POSITION:		DATE:	

CHILDMINDING ACCIDENT/ INCIDENT REPORT

INCIDENT NO:	INCIDENT DATE:	INCIDENT TIME:
LOCATION:	REPORTED TIME:	REPORTED DATE:

| PERSON INJURED / INVOLVED | O STUDENT O ACADEMIC STAFF O NON-ACADEMIC STAFF
O VISITOR O OTHER : | |

FULLNAME:		CLASS:

ADDRESS:

NATURE & EXTENT OF INJURIES	O GRAZE O BUMP O CUT O FALL O NOSEBLEED O SCRATCHES O OTHER:

DETAILS OF INCIDENT / ACCIDENT

WHAT ACTION WAS TAKEN ?	O FIRST AID O AMBULLANCE CALLED O HOSPITAL O POLICE O OTHER:

WITNESS (ES)	ACTION (S) WHICH COULD HAVE PREVENTED THE INCIDENT
1.	
2.	
3.	

EMERGENCY CONTACT (PARENT / GUARDIAN INFORMATION)

FULLNAME:		
E-MAIL ADDRESS:		PHONE No:
OUTCOME	O PARENT SPOKEN TO O VOICEMAIL O NO ANSWER	
CONTACT MADE BY:		TIME:
INCIDENT HANDLED BY:		
TREATMENT GIVEN BY:		
FORM COMPLETED BY:		
POSITION:		DATE:
APPROVED BY:		
POSITION:		DATE:

CHILDMINDING ACCIDENT/ INCIDENT REPORT

INCIDENT NO:	INCIDENT DATE:	INCIDENT TIME:
LOCATION:	REPORTED TIME:	REPORTED DATE:

| PERSON INJURED / INVOLVED | O STUDENT   O ACADEMIC STAFF   O NON-ACADEMIC STAFF
O VISITOR   O OTHER : | |

FULLNAME:		CLASS:

ADDRESS:		

| NATURE & EXTENT OF INJURIES | O GRAZE   O BUMP   O CUT   O FALL   O NOSEBLEED
O SCRATCHES   O OTHER: | |

DETAILS OF INCIDENT / ACCIDENT

WHAT ACTION WAS TAKEN ?	O FIRST AID O AMBULLANCE CALLED O HOSPITAL O POLICE O OTHER:

WITNESS (ES)	ACTION (S) WHICH COULD HAVE PREVENTED THE INCIDENT
1.	
2.	
3.	

EMERGENCY CONTACT (PARENT / GUARDIAN INFORMATION)

FULLNAME:		
E-MAIL ADDRESS:		PHONE No:
OUTCOME	O PARENT SPOKEN TO O VOICEMAIL	O NO ANSWER
CONTACT MADE BY:		TIME:
INCIDENT HANDLED BY:		
TREATMENT GIVEN BY:		
FORM COMPLETED BY:		
POSITION:		DATE:
APPROVED BY:		
POSITION:		DATE:

CHILDMINDING ACCIDENT/ INCIDENT REPORT

INCIDENT NO:	INCIDENT DATE:		INCIDENT TIME:
LOCATION:	REPORTED TIME:		REPORTED DATE:
PERSON INJURED / INVOLVED	O STUDENT　　O ACADEMIC STAFF　　O NON-ACADEMIC STAFF O VISITOR　　O OTHER :		
FULLNAME:		CLASS:	
ADDRESS:			
NATURE & EXTENT OF INJURIES	O GRAZE　　O BUMP　　O CUT　　O FALL　　O NOSEBLEED O SCRATCHES　　O OTHER:		

DETAILS OF INCIDENT / ACCIDENT

WHAT ACTION WAS TAKEN ?	O FIRST AID　　O AMBULLANCE CALLED　　O HOSPITAL　　O POLICE O OTHER:

WITNESS (ES)	ACTION (S) WHICH COULD HAVE PREVENTED THE INCIDENT
1.	
2.	
3.	

EMERGENCY CONTACT (PARENT / GUARDIAN INFORMATION)

FULLNAME:			
E-MAIL ADDRESS:		PHONE No:	
OUTCOME	O PARENT SPOKEN TO	O VOICEMAIL	O NO ANSWER
CONTACT MADE BY:		TIME:	
INCIDENT HANDLED BY:			
TREATMENT GIVEN BY:			
FORM COMPLETED BY:			
POSITION:		DATE:	
APPROVED BY:			
POSITION:		DATE:	

CHILDMINDING ACCIDENT/ INCIDENT REPORT

INCIDENT NO:	INCIDENT DATE:	INCIDENT TIME:
LOCATION:	REPORTED TIME:	REPORTED DATE:

| PERSON INJURED / INVOLVED | O STUDENT   O ACADEMIC STAFF   O NON-ACADEMIC STAFF
 O VISITOR   O OTHER : | | |

FULLNAME:		CLASS:

ADDRESS:		

NATURE & EXTENT OF INJURIES	O GRAZE O BUMP O CUT O FALL O NOSEBLEED O SCRATCHES O OTHER:

DETAILS OF INCIDENT / ACCIDENT

WHAT ACTION WAS TAKEN ?	O FIRST AID O AMBULLANCE CALLED O HOSPITAL O POLICE O OTHER:

WITNESS (ES)	ACTION (S) WHICH COULD HAVE PREVENTED THE INCIDENT
1.	
2.	
3.	

EMERGENCY CONTACT (PARENT / GUARDIAN INFORMATION)

FULLNAME:		
E-MAIL ADDRESS:		PHONE No:
OUTCOME	O PARENT SPOKEN TO O VOICEMAIL	O NO ANSWER
CONTACT MADE BY:		TIME:
INCIDENT HANDLED BY:		
TREATMENT GIVEN BY:		
FORM COMPLETED BY:		
POSITION:		DATE:
APPROVED BY:		
POSITION:		DATE:

CHILDMINDING ACCIDENT/ INCIDENT REPORT

INCIDENT NO:	INCIDENT DATE:	INCIDENT TIME:
LOCATION:	REPORTED TIME:	REPORTED DATE:

PERSON INJURED / INVOLVED	O STUDENT O ACADEMIC STAFF O NON-ACADEMIC STAFF O VISITOR O OTHER :	

FULLNAME:		CLASS:

ADDRESS:	

NATURE & EXTENT OF INJURIES	O GRAZE O BUMP O CUT O FALL O NOSEBLEED O SCRATCHES O OTHER:

DETAILS OF INCIDENT / ACCIDENT

WHAT ACTION WAS TAKEN ?	O FIRST AID O AMBULLANCE CALLED O HOSPITAL O POLICE O OTHER:

WITNESS (ES)	ACTION (S) WHICH COULD HAVE PREVENTED THE INCIDENT
1.	
2.	
3.	

EMERGENCY CONTACT (PARENT / GUARDIAN INFORMATION)

FULLNAME:	
E-MAIL ADDRESS:	PHONE No:
OUTCOME O PARENT SPOKEN TO O VOICEMAIL O NO ANSWER	
CONTACT MADE BY:	TIME:
INCIDENT HANDLED BY:	
TREATMENT GIVEN BY:	
FORM COMPLETED BY:	
POSITION:	DATE:
APPROVED BY:	
POSITION:	DATE:

CHILDMINDING ACCIDENT/ INCIDENT REPORT

INCIDENT NO:	INCIDENT DATE:		INCIDENT TIME:
LOCATION:	REPORTED TIME:		REPORTED DATE:
PERSON INJURED / INVOLVED	○ STUDENT ○ ACADEMIC STAFF ○ NON-ACADEMIC STAFF ○ VISITOR ○ OTHER :		
FULLNAME:		CLASS:	
ADDRESS:			
NATURE & EXTENT OF INJURIES	○ GRAZE ○ BUMP ○ CUT ○ FALL ○ NOSEBLEED ○ SCRATCHES ○ OTHER:		

DETAILS OF INCIDENT / ACCIDENT

WHAT ACTION WAS TAKEN ?	○ FIRST AID ○ AMBULLANCE CALLED ○ HOSPITAL ○ POLICE ○ OTHER:

WITNESS (ES)	ACTION (S) WHICH COULD HAVE PREVENTED THE INCIDENT
1.	
2.	
3.	

EMERGENCY CONTACT (PARENT / GUARDIAN INFORMATION)

FULLNAME:			
E-MAIL ADDRESS:		PHONE No:	
OUTCOME	○ PARENT SPOKEN TO	○ VOICEMAIL	○ NO ANSWER
CONTACT MADE BY:		TIME:	
INCIDENT HANDLED BY:			
TREATMENT GIVEN BY:			
FORM COMPLETED BY:			
POSITION:		DATE:	
APPROVED BY:			
POSITION:		DATE:	

CHILDMINDING ACCIDENT/ INCIDENT REPORT

INCIDENT NO:	INCIDENT DATE:	INCIDENT TIME:
LOCATION:	REPORTED TIME:	REPORTED DATE:

| PERSON INJURED / INVOLVED | O STUDENT   O ACADEMIC STAFF   O NON-ACADEMIC STAFF
 O VISITOR   O OTHER : | |

FULLNAME:		CLASS:

ADDRESS:		

| NATURE & EXTENT OF INJURIES | O GRAZE   O BUMP   O CUT   O FALL   O NOSEBLEED
 O SCRATCHES   O OTHER: | |

DETAILS OF INCIDENT / ACCIDENT

WHAT ACTION WAS TAKEN ?	O FIRST AID O AMBULLANCE CALLED O HOSPITAL O POLICE O OTHER:

WITNESS (ES)	ACTION (S) WHICH COULD HAVE PREVENTED THE INCIDENT
1.	
2.	
3.	

EMERGENCY CONTACT (PARENT / GUARDIAN INFORMATION)

FULLNAME:		
E-MAIL ADDRESS:		PHONE No:
OUTCOME	O PARENT SPOKEN TO O VOICEMAIL O NO ANSWER	
CONTACT MADE BY:		TIME:
INCIDENT HANDLED BY:		
TREATMENT GIVEN BY:		
FORM COMPLETED BY:		
POSITION:		DATE:
APPROVED BY:		
POSITION:		DATE:

CHILDMINDING ACCIDENT/ INCIDENT REPORT

INCIDENT NO:	INCIDENT DATE:	INCIDENT TIME:
LOCATION:	REPORTED TIME:	REPORTED DATE:

| PERSON INJURED / INVOLVED | O STUDENT   O ACADEMIC STAFF   O NON-ACADEMIC STAFF
O VISITOR   O OTHER : | | |

FULLNAME:	CLASS:

ADDRESS:	

NATURE & EXTENT OF INJURIES	O GRAZE O BUMP O CUT O FALL O NOSEBLEED O SCRATCHES O OTHER:

DETAILS OF INCIDENT / ACCIDENT

WHAT ACTION WAS TAKEN ?	O FIRST AID O AMBULLANCE CALLED O HOSPITAL O POLICE O OTHER:

WITNESS (ES)	ACTION (S) WHICH COULD HAVE PREVENTED THE INCIDENT
1.	
2.	
3.	

EMERGENCY CONTACT (PARENT / GUARDIAN INFORMATION)

FULLNAME:	
E-MAIL ADDRESS:	PHONE No:
OUTCOME	O PARENT SPOKEN TO O VOICEMAIL O NO ANSWER
CONTACT MADE BY:	TIME:
INCIDENT HANDLED BY:	
TREATMENT GIVEN BY:	
FORM COMPLETED BY:	
POSITION:	DATE:
APPROVED BY:	
POSITION:	DATE:

CHILDMINDING ACCIDENT/ INCIDENT REPORT

INCIDENT NO:	INCIDENT DATE:	INCIDENT TIME:
LOCATION:	REPORTED TIME:	REPORTED DATE:

PERSON INJURED / INVOLVED	O STUDENT O ACADEMIC STAFF O NON-ACADEMIC STAFF O VISITOR O OTHER :	

FULLNAME:		CLASS:

ADDRESS:		

NATURE & EXTENT OF INJURIES	O GRAZE O BUMP O CUT O FALL O NOSEBLEED O SCRATCHES O OTHER:	

DETAILS OF INCIDENT / ACCIDENT

WHAT ACTION WAS TAKEN ?	O FIRST AID O AMBULLANCE CALLED O HOSPITAL O POLICE O OTHER:

WITNESS (ES)	ACTION (S) WHICH COULD HAVE PREVENTED THE INCIDENT
1.	
2.	
3.	

EMERGENCY CONTACT (PARENT / GUARDIAN INFORMATION)

FULLNAME:		
E-MAIL ADDRESS:		PHONE No:
OUTCOME	O PARENT SPOKEN TO O VOICEMAIL O NO ANSWER	
CONTACT MADE BY:		TIME:
INCIDENT HANDLED BY:		
TREATMENT GIVEN BY:		
FORM COMPLETED BY:		
POSITION:		DATE:
APPROVED BY:		
POSITION:		DATE:

CHILDMINDING ACCIDENT/ INCIDENT REPORT

INCIDENT NO:	INCIDENT DATE:	INCIDENT TIME:
LOCATION:	REPORTED TIME:	REPORTED DATE:

PERSON INJURED / INVOLVED	○ STUDENT ○ ACADEMIC STAFF ○ NON-ACADEMIC STAFF ○ VISITOR ○ OTHER :

FULLNAME:	CLASS:

ADDRESS:

NATURE & EXTENT OF INJURIES	○ GRAZE ○ BUMP ○ CUT ○ FALL ○ NOSEBLEED ○ SCRATCHES ○ OTHER:

DETAILS OF INCIDENT / ACCIDENT

WHAT ACTION WAS TAKEN ?	○ FIRST AID ○ AMBULLANCE CALLED ○ HOSPITAL ○ POLICE ○ OTHER:

WITNESS (ES)	ACTION (S) WHICH COULD HAVE PREVENTED THE INCIDENT
1.	
2.	
3.	

EMERGENCY CONTACT (PARENT / GUARDIAN INFORMATION)

FULLNAME:		
E-MAIL ADDRESS:		PHONE No:
OUTCOME	○ PARENT SPOKEN TO ○ VOICEMAIL	○ NO ANSWER
CONTACT MADE BY:		TIME:
INCIDENT HANDLED BY:		
TREATMENT GIVEN BY:		
FORM COMPLETED BY:		
POSITION:		DATE:
APPROVED BY:		
POSITION:		DATE:

CHILDMINDING ACCIDENT/ INCIDENT REPORT

INCIDENT NO:	INCIDENT DATE:	INCIDENT TIME:
LOCATION:	REPORTED TIME:	REPORTED DATE:

PERSON INJURED / INVOLVED	○ STUDENT ○ ACADEMIC STAFF ○ NON-ACADEMIC STAFF ○ VISITOR ○ OTHER :

FULLNAME:	CLASS:

ADDRESS:

NATURE & EXTENT OF INJURIES	○ GRAZE ○ BUMP ○ CUT ○ FALL ○ NOSEBLEED ○ SCRATCHES ○ OTHER:

DETAILS OF INCIDENT / ACCIDENT

WHAT ACTION WAS TAKEN ?	○ FIRST AID ○ AMBULLANCE CALLED ○ HOSPITAL ○ POLICE ○ OTHER:

WITNESS (ES)	ACTION (S) WHICH COULD HAVE PREVENTED THE INCIDENT
1.	
2.	
3.	

EMERGENCY CONTACT (PARENT / GUARDIAN INFORMATION)

FULLNAME:		
E-MAIL ADDRESS:	PHONE No:	
OUTCOME	○ PARENT SPOKEN TO ○ VOICEMAIL ○ NO ANSWER	
CONTACT MADE BY:	TIME:	
INCIDENT HANDLED BY:		
TREATMENT GIVEN BY:		
FORM COMPLETED BY:		
POSITION:	DATE:	
APPROVED BY:		
POSITION:	DATE:	

CHILDMINDING ACCIDENT/ INCIDENT REPORT

INCIDENT NO:	INCIDENT DATE:	INCIDENT TIME:
LOCATION:	REPORTED TIME:	REPORTED DATE:

PERSON INJURED / INVOLVED	O STUDENT O ACADEMIC STAFF O NON-ACADEMIC STAFF O VISITOR O OTHER :

FULLNAME:		CLASS:
ADDRESS:		

NATURE & EXTENT OF INJURIES	O GRAZE O BUMP O CUT O FALL O NOSEBLEED O SCRATCHES O OTHER:

DETAILS OF INCIDENT / ACCIDENT

WHAT ACTION WAS TAKEN ?	O FIRST AID O AMBULLANCE CALLED O HOSPITAL O POLICE O OTHER:

WITNESS (ES)	ACTION (S) WHICH COULD HAVE PREVENTED THE INCIDENT
1.	
2.	
3.	

EMERGENCY CONTACT (PARENT / GUARDIAN INFORMATION)

FULLNAME:		
E-MAIL ADDRESS:		PHONE No:
OUTCOME	O PARENT SPOKEN TO O VOICEMAIL O NO ANSWER	
CONTACT MADE BY:		TIME:
INCIDENT HANDLED BY:		
TREATMENT GIVEN BY:		
FORM COMPLETED BY:		
POSITION:		DATE:
APPROVED BY:		
POSITION:		DATE:

CHILDMINDING ACCIDENT/ INCIDENT REPORT

INCIDENT NO:	INCIDENT DATE:	INCIDENT TIME:
LOCATION:	REPORTED TIME:	REPORTED DATE:

PERSON INJURED / INVOLVED	○ STUDENT ○ ACADEMIC STAFF ○ NON-ACADEMIC STAFF ○ VISITOR ○ OTHER :		

FULLNAME:		CLASS:

ADDRESS:		

NATURE & EXTENT OF INJURIES	○ GRAZE ○ BUMP ○ CUT ○ FALL ○ NOSEBLEED ○ SCRATCHES ○ OTHER:

DETAILS OF INCIDENT / ACCIDENT

WHAT ACTION WAS TAKEN ?	○ FIRST AID ○ AMBULLANCE CALLED ○ HOSPITAL ○ POLICE ○ OTHER:

WITNESS (ES)	ACTION (S) WHICH COULD HAVE PREVENTED THE INCIDENT
1.	
2.	
3.	

EMERGENCY CONTACT (PARENT / GUARDIAN INFORMATION)

FULLNAME:		
E-MAIL ADDRESS:		PHONE No:
OUTCOME	○ PARENT SPOKEN TO	○ VOICEMAIL ○ NO ANSWER
CONTACT MADE BY:		TIME:
INCIDENT HANDLED BY:		
TREATMENT GIVEN BY:		
FORM COMPLETED BY:		
POSITION:		DATE:
APPROVED BY:		
POSITION:		DATE:

CHILDMINDING ACCIDENT/ INCIDENT REPORT

INCIDENT NO:	INCIDENT DATE:	INCIDENT TIME:
LOCATION:	REPORTED TIME:	REPORTED DATE:

PERSON INJURED / INVOLVED	O STUDENT O ACADEMIC STAFF O NON-ACADEMIC STAFF O VISITOR O OTHER :

FULLNAME:	CLASS:

ADDRESS:

NATURE & EXTENT OF INJURIES	O GRAZE O BUMP O CUT O FALL O NOSEBLEED O SCRATCHES O OTHER:

DETAILS OF INCIDENT / ACCIDENT

WHAT ACTION WAS TAKEN ?	O FIRST AID O AMBULLANCE CALLED O HOSPITAL O POLICE O OTHER:

WITNESS (ES)	ACTION (S) WHICH COULD HAVE PREVENTED THE INCIDENT
1.	
2.	
3.	

EMERGENCY CONTACT (PARENT / GUARDIAN INFORMATION)

FULLNAME:		
E-MAIL ADDRESS:		PHONE No:
OUTCOME	O PARENT SPOKEN TO O VOICEMAIL O NO ANSWER	
CONTACT MADE BY:		TIME:
INCIDENT HANDLED BY:		
TREATMENT GIVEN BY:		
FORM COMPLETED BY:		
POSITION:		DATE:
APPROVED BY:		
POSITION:		DATE:

CHILDMINDING ACCIDENT/ INCIDENT REPORT

INCIDENT NO:	INCIDENT DATE:	INCIDENT TIME:
LOCATION:	REPORTED TIME:	REPORTED DATE:

PERSON INJURED / INVOLVED	○ STUDENT ○ ACADEMIC STAFF ○ NON-ACADEMIC STAFF ○ VISITOR ○ OTHER :

FULLNAME:	CLASS:

ADDRESS:

NATURE & EXTENT OF INJURIES	○ GRAZE ○ BUMP ○ CUT ○ FALL ○ NOSEBLEED ○ SCRATCHES ○ OTHER:

DETAILS OF INCIDENT / ACCIDENT

WHAT ACTION WAS TAKEN ?	○ FIRST AID ○ AMBULLANCE CALLED ○ HOSPITAL ○ POLICE ○ OTHER:

WITNESS (ES)	ACTION (S) WHICH COULD HAVE PREVENTED THE INCIDENT
1.	
2.	
3.	

EMERGENCY CONTACT (PARENT / GUARDIAN INFORMATION)

FULLNAME:	
E-MAIL ADDRESS:	PHONE No:
OUTCOME	○ PARENT SPOKEN TO ○ VOICEMAIL ○ NO ANSWER
CONTACT MADE BY:	TIME:
INCIDENT HANDLED BY:	
TREATMENT GIVEN BY:	
FORM COMPLETED BY:	
POSITION:	DATE:
APPROVED BY:	
POSITION:	DATE:

CHILDMINDING ACCIDENT/ INCIDENT REPORT

INCIDENT NO:	INCIDENT DATE:	INCIDENT TIME:
LOCATION:	REPORTED TIME:	REPORTED DATE:

PERSON INJURED / INVOLVED	O STUDENT O ACADEMIC STAFF O NON-ACADEMIC STAFF O VISITOR O OTHER :

FULLNAME:	CLASS:

ADDRESS:	

NATURE & EXTENT OF INJURIES	O GRAZE O BUMP O CUT O FALL O NOSEBLEED O SCRATCHES O OTHER:

DETAILS OF INCIDENT / ACCIDENT

WHAT ACTION WAS TAKEN ?	O FIRST AID O AMBULLANCE CALLED O HOSPITAL O POLICE O OTHER:

WITNESS (ES)	ACTION (S) WHICH COULD HAVE PREVENTED THE INCIDENT
1.	
2.	
3.	

EMERGENCY CONTACT (PARENT / GUARDIAN INFORMATION)

FULLNAME:	
E-MAIL ADDRESS:	PHONE No:
OUTCOME O PARENT SPOKEN TO O VOICEMAIL O NO ANSWER	
CONTACT MADE BY:	TIME:
INCIDENT HANDLED BY:	
TREATMENT GIVEN BY:	
FORM COMPLETED BY:	
POSITION:	DATE:
APPROVED BY:	
POSITION:	DATE:

CHILDMINDING ACCIDENT/ INCIDENT REPORT

INCIDENT NO:	INCIDENT DATE:	INCIDENT TIME:
LOCATION:	REPORTED TIME:	REPORTED DATE:

PERSON INJURED / INVOLVED	O STUDENT O ACADEMIC STAFF O NON-ACADEMIC STAFF O VISITOR O OTHER :	
FULLNAME:		CLASS:
ADDRESS:		
NATURE & EXTENT OF INJURIES	O GRAZE O BUMP O CUT O FALL O NOSEBLEED O SCRATCHES O OTHER:	

DETAILS OF INCIDENT / ACCIDENT

WHAT ACTION WAS TAKEN ?	O FIRST AID O AMBULLANCE CALLED O HOSPITAL O POLICE O OTHER:

WITNESS (ES)	ACTION (S) WHICH COULD HAVE PREVENTED THE INCIDENT
1.	
2.	
3.	

EMERGENCY CONTACT (PARENT / GUARDIAN INFORMATION)

FULLNAME:		
E-MAIL ADDRESS:		PHONE No:
OUTCOME	O PARENT SPOKEN TO O VOICEMAIL	O NO ANSWER
CONTACT MADE BY:		TIME:
INCIDENT HANDLED BY:		
TREATMENT GIVEN BY:		
FORM COMPLETED BY:		
POSITION:		DATE:
APPROVED BY:		
POSITION:		DATE:

CHILDMINDING ACCIDENT/ INCIDENT REPORT

INCIDENT NO:	INCIDENT DATE:	INCIDENT TIME:
LOCATION:	REPORTED TIME:	REPORTED DATE:

PERSON INJURED / INVOLVED	○ STUDENT ○ ACADEMIC STAFF ○ NON-ACADEMIC STAFF ○ VISITOR ○ OTHER :

FULLNAME:	CLASS:

ADDRESS:	

NATURE & EXTENT OF INJURIES	○ GRAZE ○ BUMP ○ CUT ○ FALL ○ NOSEBLEED ○ SCRATCHES ○ OTHER:

DETAILS OF INCIDENT / ACCIDENT

WHAT ACTION WAS TAKEN ?	○ FIRST AID ○ AMBULLANCE CALLED ○ HOSPITAL ○ POLICE ○ OTHER:

WITNESS (ES)	ACTION (S) WHICH COULD HAVE PREVENTED THE INCIDENT
1.	
2.	
3.	

EMERGENCY CONTACT (PARENT / GUARDIAN INFORMATION)

FULLNAME:		
E-MAIL ADDRESS:	PHONE No:	
OUTCOME	○ PARENT SPOKEN TO ○ VOICEMAIL ○ NO ANSWER	
CONTACT MADE BY:	TIME:	
INCIDENT HANDLED BY:		
TREATMENT GIVEN BY:		
FORM COMPLETED BY:		
POSITION:	DATE:	
APPROVED BY:		
POSITION:	DATE:	

CHILDMINDING ACCIDENT/ INCIDENT REPORT

INCIDENT NO:	INCIDENT DATE:	INCIDENT TIME:
LOCATION:	REPORTED TIME:	REPORTED DATE:

| PERSON INJURED / INVOLVED | ○ STUDENT ○ ACADEMIC STAFF ○ NON-ACADEMIC STAFF ○ VISITOR ○ OTHER : |||

FULLNAME:		CLASS:
ADDRESS:		

| NATURE & EXTENT OF INJURIES | ○ GRAZE ○ BUMP ○ CUT ○ FALL ○ NOSEBLEED ○ SCRATCHES ○ OTHER: |

DETAILS OF INCIDENT / ACCIDENT

WHAT ACTION WAS TAKEN ?	○ FIRST AID ○ AMBULLANCE CALLED ○ HOSPITAL ○ POLICE ○ OTHER:

WITNESS (ES)	ACTION (S) WHICH COULD HAVE PREVENTED THE INCIDENT
1.	
2.	
3.	

EMERGENCY CONTACT (PARENT / GUARDIAN INFORMATION)

FULLNAME:		
E-MAIL ADDRESS:	PHONE No:	
OUTCOME	○ PARENT SPOKEN TO ○ VOICEMAIL ○ NO ANSWER	
CONTACT MADE BY:	TIME:	
INCIDENT HANDLED BY:		
TREATMENT GIVEN BY:		
FORM COMPLETED BY:		
POSITION:	DATE:	
APPROVED BY:		
POSITION:	DATE:	

CHILDMINDING ACCIDENT/ INCIDENT REPORT

INCIDENT NO:	INCIDENT DATE:	INCIDENT TIME:
LOCATION:	REPORTED TIME:	REPORTED DATE:

PERSON INJURED / INVOLVED	○ STUDENT ○ ACADEMIC STAFF ○ NON-ACADEMIC STAFF ○ VISITOR ○ OTHER :

FULLNAME:	CLASS:

ADDRESS:

NATURE & EXTENT OF INJURIES	○ GRAZE ○ BUMP ○ CUT ○ FALL ○ NOSEBLEED ○ SCRATCHES ○ OTHER:

DETAILS OF INCIDENT / ACCIDENT

WHAT ACTION WAS TAKEN ?	○ FIRST AID ○ AMBULLANCE CALLED ○ HOSPITAL ○ POLICE ○ OTHER:

WITNESS (ES)	ACTION (S) WHICH COULD HAVE PREVENTED THE INCIDENT
1.	
2.	
3.	

EMERGENCY CONTACT (PARENT / GUARDIAN INFORMATION)

FULLNAME:		
E-MAIL ADDRESS:	PHONE No:	
OUTCOME	○ PARENT SPOKEN TO ○ VOICEMAIL	○ NO ANSWER
CONTACT MADE BY:	TIME:	
INCIDENT HANDLED BY:		
TREATMENT GIVEN BY:		
FORM COMPLETED BY:		
POSITION:	DATE:	
APPROVED BY:		
POSITION:	DATE:	

CHILDMINDING ACCIDENT/ INCIDENT REPORT

INCIDENT NO:	INCIDENT DATE:	INCIDENT TIME:
LOCATION:	REPORTED TIME:	REPORTED DATE:

PERSON INJURED / INVOLVED	○ STUDENT ○ ACADEMIC STAFF ○ NON-ACADEMIC STAFF ○ VISITOR ○ OTHER :

FULLNAME:	CLASS:

ADDRESS:

NATURE & EXTENT OF INJURIES	○ GRAZE ○ BUMP ○ CUT ○ FALL ○ NOSEBLEED ○ SCRATCHES ○ OTHER:

DETAILS OF INCIDENT / ACCIDENT

WHAT ACTION WAS TAKEN ?	○ FIRST AID ○ AMBULLANCE CALLED ○ HOSPITAL ○ POLICE ○ OTHER:

WITNESS (ES)	ACTION (S) WHICH COULD HAVE PREVENTED THE INCIDENT
1.	
2.	
3.	

EMERGENCY CONTACT (PARENT / GUARDIAN INFORMATION)

FULLNAME:		
E-MAIL ADDRESS:	PHONE No:	
OUTCOME	○ PARENT SPOKEN TO ○ VOICEMAIL ○ NO ANSWER	
CONTACT MADE BY:	TIME:	
INCIDENT HANDLED BY:		
TREATMENT GIVEN BY:		
FORM COMPLETED BY:		
POSITION:	DATE:	
APPROVED BY:		
POSITION:	DATE:	

CHILDMINDING ACCIDENT/ INCIDENT REPORT

INCIDENT NO:	INCIDENT DATE:	INCIDENT TIME:
LOCATION:	REPORTED TIME:	REPORTED DATE:

PERSON INJURED / INVOLVED	O STUDENT O ACADEMIC STAFF O NON-ACADEMIC STAFF O VISITOR O OTHER :

FULLNAME:	CLASS:

ADDRESS:	

NATURE & EXTENT OF INJURIES	O GRAZE O BUMP O CUT O FALL O NOSEBLEED O SCRATCHES O OTHER:

DETAILS OF INCIDENT / ACCIDENT

WHAT ACTION WAS TAKEN ?	O FIRST AID O AMBULLANCE CALLED O HOSPITAL O POLICE O OTHER:

WITNESS (ES)	ACTION (S) WHICH COULD HAVE PREVENTED THE INCIDENT
1.	
2.	
3.	

EMERGENCY CONTACT (PARENT / GUARDIAN INFORMATION)

FULLNAME:		
E-MAIL ADDRESS:	PHONE No:	
OUTCOME	O PARENT SPOKEN TO O VOICEMAIL O NO ANSWER	
CONTACT MADE BY:	TIME:	
INCIDENT HANDLED BY:		
TREATMENT GIVEN BY:		
FORM COMPLETED BY:		
POSITION:	DATE:	
APPROVED BY:		
POSITION:	DATE:	

CHILDMINDING ACCIDENT/ INCIDENT REPORT

INCIDENT NO:	INCIDENT DATE:	INCIDENT TIME:
LOCATION:	REPORTED TIME:	REPORTED DATE:

PERSON INJURED / INVOLVED	○ STUDENT ○ ACADEMIC STAFF ○ NON-ACADEMIC STAFF ○ VISITOR ○ OTHER :

FULLNAME:	CLASS:

ADDRESS:	

NATURE & EXTENT OF INJURIES	○ GRAZE ○ BUMP ○ CUT ○ FALL ○ NOSEBLEED ○ SCRATCHES ○ OTHER:

DETAILS OF INCIDENT / ACCIDENT

WHAT ACTION WAS TAKEN ?	○ FIRST AID ○ AMBULLANCE CALLED ○ HOSPITAL ○ POLICE ○ OTHER:

WITNESS (ES)	ACTION (S) WHICH COULD HAVE PREVENTED THE INCIDENT
1.	
2.	
3.	

EMERGENCY CONTACT (PARENT / GUARDIAN INFORMATION)

FULLNAME:		
E-MAIL ADDRESS:	PHONE No:	
OUTCOME	○ PARENT SPOKEN TO ○ VOICEMAIL ○ NO ANSWER	
CONTACT MADE BY:	TIME:	
INCIDENT HANDLED BY:		
TREATMENT GIVEN BY:		
FORM COMPLETED BY:		
POSITION:	DATE:	
APPROVED BY:		
POSITION:	DATE:	

CHILDMINDING ACCIDENT/ INCIDENT REPORT

INCIDENT NO:	INCIDENT DATE:	INCIDENT TIME:
LOCATION:	REPORTED TIME:	REPORTED DATE:

PERSON INJURED / INVOLVED	○ STUDENT ○ ACADEMIC STAFF ○ NON-ACADEMIC STAFF ○ VISITOR ○ OTHER :

FULLNAME:	CLASS:

ADDRESS:	

NATURE & EXTENT OF INJURIES	○ GRAZE ○ BUMP ○ CUT ○ FALL ○ NOSEBLEED ○ SCRATCHES ○ OTHER:

DETAILS OF INCIDENT / ACCIDENT

WHAT ACTION WAS TAKEN ?	○ FIRST AID ○ AMBULLANCE CALLED ○ HOSPITAL ○ POLICE ○ OTHER:

WITNESS (ES)	ACTION (S) WHICH COULD HAVE PREVENTED THE INCIDENT
1.	
2.	
3.	

EMERGENCY CONTACT (PARENT / GUARDIAN INFORMATION)

FULLNAME:	
E-MAIL ADDRESS:	PHONE No:
OUTCOME	○ PARENT SPOKEN TO ○ VOICEMAIL ○ NO ANSWER
CONTACT MADE BY:	TIME:
INCIDENT HANDLED BY:	
TREATMENT GIVEN BY:	
FORM COMPLETED BY:	
POSITION:	DATE:
APPROVED BY:	
POSITION:	DATE:

CHILDMINDING ACCIDENT/ INCIDENT REPORT

INCIDENT NO:	INCIDENT DATE:	INCIDENT TIME:
LOCATION:	REPORTED TIME:	REPORTED DATE:

| PERSON INJURED / INVOLVED | ○ STUDENT ○ ACADEMIC STAFF ○ NON-ACADEMIC STAFF ○ VISITOR ○ OTHER : | |

FULLNAME:		CLASS:

ADDRESS:

NATURE & EXTENT OF INJURIES	○ GRAZE ○ BUMP ○ CUT ○ FALL ○ NOSEBLEED ○ SCRATCHES ○ OTHER:

DETAILS OF INCIDENT / ACCIDENT

WHAT ACTION WAS TAKEN ?	○ FIRST AID ○ AMBULLANCE CALLED ○ HOSPITAL ○ POLICE ○ OTHER:

WITNESS (ES)	ACTION (S) WHICH COULD HAVE PREVENTED THE INCIDENT
1.	
2.	
3.	

EMERGENCY CONTACT (PARENT / GUARDIAN INFORMATION)

FULLNAME:		
E-MAIL ADDRESS:		PHONE No:
OUTCOME	○ PARENT SPOKEN TO ○ VOICEMAIL ○ NO ANSWER	
CONTACT MADE BY:		TIME:
INCIDENT HANDLED BY:		
TREATMENT GIVEN BY:		
FORM COMPLETED BY:		
POSITION:		DATE:
APPROVED BY:		
POSITION:		DATE:

CHILDMINDING ACCIDENT/ INCIDENT REPORT

INCIDENT NO:	INCIDENT DATE:	INCIDENT TIME:
LOCATION:	REPORTED TIME:	REPORTED DATE:

PERSON INJURED / INVOLVED	O STUDENT O ACADEMIC STAFF O NON-ACADEMIC STAFF O VISITOR O OTHER :

FULLNAME:		CLASS:
ADDRESS:		

NATURE & EXTENT OF INJURIES	O GRAZE O BUMP O CUT O FALL O NOSEBLEED O SCRATCHES O OTHER:

DETAILS OF INCIDENT / ACCIDENT

WHAT ACTION WAS TAKEN ?	O FIRST AID O AMBULLANCE CALLED O HOSPITAL O POLICE O OTHER:

WITNESS (ES)	ACTION (S) WHICH COULD HAVE PREVENTED THE INCIDENT
1.	
2.	
3.	

EMERGENCY CONTACT (PARENT / GUARDIAN INFORMATION)

FULLNAME:		
E-MAIL ADDRESS:		PHONE No:
OUTCOME	O PARENT SPOKEN TO O VOICEMAIL O NO ANSWER	
CONTACT MADE BY:		TIME:
INCIDENT HANDLED BY:		
TREATMENT GIVEN BY:		
FORM COMPLETED BY:		
POSITION:		DATE:
APPROVED BY:		
POSITION:		DATE:

CHILDMINDING ACCIDENT/ INCIDENT REPORT

INCIDENT NO:	INCIDENT DATE:	INCIDENT TIME:
LOCATION:	REPORTED TIME:	REPORTED DATE:

PERSON INJURED / INVOLVED	O STUDENT O ACADEMIC STAFF O NON-ACADEMIC STAFF O VISITOR O OTHER :

FULLNAME:	CLASS:

ADDRESS:

NATURE & EXTENT OF INJURIES	O GRAZE O BUMP O CUT O FALL O NOSEBLEED O SCRATCHES O OTHER:

DETAILS OF INCIDENT / ACCIDENT

WHAT ACTION WAS TAKEN ?	O FIRST AID O AMBULLANCE CALLED O HOSPITAL O POLICE O OTHER:

WITNESS (ES)	ACTION (S) WHICH COULD HAVE PREVENTED THE INCIDENT
1.	
2.	
3.	

EMERGENCY CONTACT (PARENT / GUARDIAN INFORMATION)

FULLNAME:	
E-MAIL ADDRESS:	PHONE No:
OUTCOME O PARENT SPOKEN TO O VOICEMAIL O NO ANSWER	
CONTACT MADE BY:	TIME:
INCIDENT HANDLED BY:	
TREATMENT GIVEN BY:	
FORM COMPLETED BY:	
POSITION:	DATE:
APPROVED BY:	
POSITION:	DATE:

CHILDMINDING ACCIDENT/ INCIDENT REPORT

INCIDENT NO:	INCIDENT DATE:	INCIDENT TIME:
LOCATION:	REPORTED TIME:	REPORTED DATE:

| PERSON INJURED / INVOLVED | O STUDENT   O ACADEMIC STAFF   O NON-ACADEMIC STAFF
O VISITOR   O OTHER : |||

FULLNAME:		CLASS:

ADDRESS:

| NATURE & EXTENT OF INJURIES | O GRAZE   O BUMP   O CUT   O FALL   O NOSEBLEED
O SCRATCHES   O OTHER: |

DETAILS OF INCIDENT / ACCIDENT

| WHAT ACTION WAS TAKEN ? | O FIRST AID   O AMBULLANCE CALLED   O HOSPITAL   O POLICE
O OTHER: |

WITNESS (ES)	ACTION (S) WHICH COULD HAVE PREVENTED THE INCIDENT
1.	
2.	
3.	

EMERGENCY CONTACT (PARENT / GUARDIAN INFORMATION)

FULLNAME:		
E-MAIL ADDRESS:		PHONE No:
OUTCOME	O PARENT SPOKEN TO O VOICEMAIL O NO ANSWER	
CONTACT MADE BY:		TIME:
INCIDENT HANDLED BY:		
TREATMENT GIVEN BY:		
FORM COMPLETED BY:		
POSITION:		DATE:
APPROVED BY:		
POSITION:		DATE:

CHILDMINDING ACCIDENT/ INCIDENT REPORT

INCIDENT NO:	INCIDENT DATE:	INCIDENT TIME:
LOCATION:	REPORTED TIME:	REPORTED DATE:

| PERSON INJURED / INVOLVED | ○ STUDENT   ○ ACADEMIC STAFF   ○ NON-ACADEMIC STAFF ○ VISITOR   ○ OTHER : | |

FULLNAME:		CLASS:

ADDRESS:		

| NATURE & EXTENT OF INJURIES | ○ GRAZE   ○ BUMP   ○ CUT   ○ FALL   ○ NOSEBLEED ○ SCRATCHES   ○ OTHER: |

DETAILS OF INCIDENT / ACCIDENT

WHAT ACTION WAS TAKEN ?	○ FIRST AID ○ AMBULLANCE CALLED ○ HOSPITAL ○ POLICE ○ OTHER:

WITNESS (ES)	ACTION (S) WHICH COULD HAVE PREVENTED THE INCIDENT
1.	
2.	
3.	

EMERGENCY CONTACT (PARENT / GUARDIAN INFORMATION)

FULLNAME:		
E-MAIL ADDRESS:		PHONE No:
OUTCOME	○ PARENT SPOKEN TO ○ VOICEMAIL ○ NO ANSWER	
CONTACT MADE BY:		TIME:
INCIDENT HANDLED BY:		
TREATMENT GIVEN BY:		
FORM COMPLETED BY:		
POSITION:		DATE:
APPROVED BY:		
POSITION:		DATE:

CHILDMINDING ACCIDENT/ INCIDENT REPORT

INCIDENT NO:	INCIDENT DATE:	INCIDENT TIME:
LOCATION:	REPORTED TIME:	REPORTED DATE:

| PERSON INJURED / INVOLVED | ○ STUDENT ○ ACADEMIC STAFF ○ NON-ACADEMIC STAFF
○ VISITOR ○ OTHER : | |

FULLNAME:		CLASS:

ADDRESS:		

| NATURE & EXTENT OF INJURIES | ○ GRAZE ○ BUMP ○ CUT ○ FALL ○ NOSEBLEED
○ SCRATCHES ○ OTHER: | |

DETAILS OF INCIDENT / ACCIDENT

| WHAT ACTION WAS TAKEN ? | ○ FIRST AID ○ AMBULLANCE CALLED ○ HOSPITAL ○ POLICE
○ OTHER: | |

WITNESS (ES)	ACTION (S) WHICH COULD HAVE PREVENTED THE INCIDENT
1.	
2.	
3.	

EMERGENCY CONTACT (PARENT / GUARDIAN INFORMATION)

FULLNAME:		
E-MAIL ADDRESS:		PHONE No:
OUTCOME	○ PARENT SPOKEN TO ○ VOICEMAIL ○ NO ANSWER	
CONTACT MADE BY:		TIME:
INCIDENT HANDLED BY:		
TREATMENT GIVEN BY:		
FORM COMPLETED BY:		
POSITION:		DATE:
APPROVED BY:		
POSITION:		DATE:

CHILDMINDING ACCIDENT/ INCIDENT REPORT

INCIDENT NO:	INCIDENT DATE:	INCIDENT TIME:
LOCATION:	REPORTED TIME:	REPORTED DATE:

PERSON INJURED / INVOLVED	O STUDENT O ACADEMIC STAFF O NON-ACADEMIC STAFF O VISITOR O OTHER :	

FULLNAME:		CLASS:

ADDRESS:		

NATURE & EXTENT OF INJURIES	O GRAZE O BUMP O CUT O FALL O NOSEBLEED O SCRATCHES O OTHER:	

DETAILS OF INCIDENT / ACCIDENT

WHAT ACTION WAS TAKEN ?	O FIRST AID O AMBULLANCE CALLED O HOSPITAL O POLICE O OTHER:

WITNESS (ES)	ACTION (S) WHICH COULD HAVE PREVENTED THE INCIDENT
1.	
2.	
3.	

EMERGENCY CONTACT (PARENT / GUARDIAN INFORMATION)

FULLNAME:		
E-MAIL ADDRESS:		PHONE No:
OUTCOME	O PARENT SPOKEN TO O VOICEMAIL O NO ANSWER	
CONTACT MADE BY:		TIME:
INCIDENT HANDLED BY:		
TREATMENT GIVEN BY:		
FORM COMPLETED BY:		
POSITION:		DATE:
APPROVED BY:		
POSITION:		DATE:

CHILDMINDING ACCIDENT/ INCIDENT REPORT

INCIDENT NO:	INCIDENT DATE:	INCIDENT TIME:
LOCATION:	REPORTED TIME:	REPORTED DATE:

PERSON INJURED / INVOLVED	○ STUDENT ○ ACADEMIC STAFF ○ NON-ACADEMIC STAFF ○ VISITOR ○ OTHER :

FULLNAME:	CLASS:

ADDRESS:

NATURE & EXTENT OF INJURIES	○ GRAZE ○ BUMP ○ CUT ○ FALL ○ NOSEBLEED ○ SCRATCHES ○ OTHER:

DETAILS OF INCIDENT / ACCIDENT

WHAT ACTION WAS TAKEN ?	○ FIRST AID ○ AMBULLANCE CALLED ○ HOSPITAL ○ POLICE ○ OTHER:

WITNESS (ES)	ACTION (S) WHICH COULD HAVE PREVENTED THE INCIDENT
1.	
2.	
3.	

EMERGENCY CONTACT (PARENT / GUARDIAN INFORMATION)

FULLNAME:	
E-MAIL ADDRESS:	PHONE No:
OUTCOME	○ PARENT SPOKEN TO ○ VOICEMAIL ○ NO ANSWER
CONTACT MADE BY:	TIME:
INCIDENT HANDLED BY:	
TREATMENT GIVEN BY:	
FORM COMPLETED BY:	
POSITION:	DATE:
APPROVED BY:	
POSITION:	DATE:

CHILDMINDING ACCIDENT/ INCIDENT REPORT

INCIDENT NO:	INCIDENT DATE:	INCIDENT TIME:
LOCATION:	REPORTED TIME:	REPORTED DATE:

PERSON INJURED / INVOLVED	O STUDENT O ACADEMIC STAFF O NON-ACADEMIC STAFF O VISITOR O OTHER :	

FULLNAME:		CLASS:

ADDRESS:		

NATURE & EXTENT OF INJURIES	O GRAZE O BUMP O CUT O FALL O NOSEBLEED O SCRATCHES O OTHER:

DETAILS OF INCIDENT / ACCIDENT

WHAT ACTION WAS TAKEN ?	O FIRST AID O AMBULLANCE CALLED O HOSPITAL O POLICE O OTHER:

WITNESS (ES)	ACTION (S) WHICH COULD HAVE PREVENTED THE INCIDENT
1.	
2.	
3.	

EMERGENCY CONTACT (PARENT / GUARDIAN INFORMATION)

FULLNAME:		
E-MAIL ADDRESS:		PHONE No:
OUTCOME	O PARENT SPOKEN TO O VOICEMAIL O NO ANSWER	
CONTACT MADE BY:		TIME:
INCIDENT HANDLED BY:		
TREATMENT GIVEN BY:		
FORM COMPLETED BY:		
POSITION:		DATE:
APPROVED BY:		
POSITION:		DATE:

CHILDMINDING ACCIDENT/ INCIDENT REPORT

INCIDENT NO:	INCIDENT DATE:	INCIDENT TIME:
LOCATION:	REPORTED TIME:	REPORTED DATE:

| PERSON INJURED / INVOLVED | ○ STUDENT ○ ACADEMIC STAFF ○ NON-ACADEMIC STAFF
○ VISITOR ○ OTHER : | |

FULLNAME:		CLASS:
ADDRESS:		

| NATURE & EXTENT OF INJURIES | ○ GRAZE ○ BUMP ○ CUT ○ FALL ○ NOSEBLEED
○ SCRATCHES ○ OTHER: |

DETAILS OF INCIDENT / ACCIDENT

| WHAT ACTION WAS TAKEN ? | ○ FIRST AID ○ AMBULLANCE CALLED ○ HOSPITAL ○ POLICE
○ OTHER: |

WITNESS (ES)	ACTION (S) WHICH COULD HAVE PREVENTED THE INCIDENT
1.	
2.	
3.	

EMERGENCY CONTACT (PARENT / GUARDIAN INFORMATION)

FULLNAME:		
E-MAIL ADDRESS:		PHONE No:
OUTCOME	○ PARENT SPOKEN TO ○ VOICEMAIL	○ NO ANSWER
CONTACT MADE BY:		TIME:
INCIDENT HANDLED BY:		
TREATMENT GIVEN BY:		
FORM COMPLETED BY:		
POSITION:		DATE:
APPROVED BY:		
POSITION:		DATE:

CHILDMINDING ACCIDENT/ INCIDENT REPORT

INCIDENT NO:	INCIDENT DATE:		INCIDENT TIME:	
LOCATION:	REPORTED TIME:		REPORTED DATE:	
PERSON INJURED / INVOLVED	○ STUDENT ○ ACADEMIC STAFF ○ NON-ACADEMIC STAFF ○ VISITOR ○ OTHER :			
FULLNAME:			CLASS:	
ADDRESS:				
NATURE & EXTENT OF INJURIES	○ GRAZE ○ BUMP ○ CUT ○ FALL ○ NOSEBLEED ○ SCRATCHES ○ OTHER:			

DETAILS OF INCIDENT / ACCIDENT

WHAT ACTION WAS TAKEN ?	○ FIRST AID ○ AMBULLANCE CALLED ○ HOSPITAL ○ POLICE ○ OTHER:

WITNESS (ES)	ACTION (S) WHICH COULD HAVE PREVENTED THE INCIDENT
1.	
2.	
3.	

EMERGENCY CONTACT (PARENT / GUARDIAN INFORMATION)

FULLNAME:		
E-MAIL ADDRESS:	PHONE No:	
OUTCOME	○ PARENT SPOKEN TO ○ VOICEMAIL	○ NO ANSWER
CONTACT MADE BY:	TIME:	
INCIDENT HANDLED BY:		
TREATMENT GIVEN BY:		
FORM COMPLETED BY:		
POSITION:	DATE:	
APPROVED BY:		
POSITION:	DATE:	

CHILDMINDING ACCIDENT/ INCIDENT REPORT

INCIDENT NO:	INCIDENT DATE:	INCIDENT TIME:
LOCATION:	REPORTED TIME:	REPORTED DATE:

PERSON INJURED / INVOLVED	O STUDENT O ACADEMIC STAFF O NON-ACADEMIC STAFF O VISITOR O OTHER :	

FULLNAME:		CLASS:

ADDRESS:		

NATURE & EXTENT OF INJURIES	O GRAZE O BUMP O CUT O FALL O NOSEBLEED O SCRATCHES O OTHER:	

DETAILS OF INCIDENT / ACCIDENT

WHAT ACTION WAS TAKEN ?	O FIRST AID O AMBULLANCE CALLED O HOSPITAL O POLICE O OTHER:

WITNESS (ES)	ACTION (S) WHICH COULD HAVE PREVENTED THE INCIDENT
1.	
2.	
3.	

EMERGENCY CONTACT (PARENT / GUARDIAN INFORMATION)

FULLNAME:		
E-MAIL ADDRESS:		PHONE No:
OUTCOME	O PARENT SPOKEN TO O VOICEMAIL	O NO ANSWER
CONTACT MADE BY:		TIME:
INCIDENT HANDLED BY:		
TREATMENT GIVEN BY:		
FORM COMPLETED BY:		
POSITION:		DATE:
APPROVED BY:		
POSITION:		DATE:

CHILDMINDING ACCIDENT/ INCIDENT REPORT

INCIDENT NO:	INCIDENT DATE:	INCIDENT TIME:
LOCATION:	REPORTED TIME:	REPORTED DATE:

| PERSON INJURED / INVOLVED | ○ STUDENT ○ ACADEMIC STAFF ○ NON-ACADEMIC STAFF ○ VISITOR ○ OTHER : |

FULLNAME:	CLASS:

ADDRESS:

| NATURE & EXTENT OF INJURIES | ○ GRAZE ○ BUMP ○ CUT ○ FALL ○ NOSEBLEED ○ SCRATCHES ○ OTHER: |

DETAILS OF INCIDENT / ACCIDENT

| WHAT ACTION WAS TAKEN ? | ○ FIRST AID ○ AMBULLANCE CALLED ○ HOSPITAL ○ POLICE ○ OTHER: |

WITNESS (ES)	ACTION (S) WHICH COULD HAVE PREVENTED THE INCIDENT
1.	
2.	
3.	

EMERGENCY CONTACT (PARENT / GUARDIAN INFORMATION)

FULLNAME:	
E-MAIL ADDRESS:	PHONE No:
OUTCOME	○ PARENT SPOKEN TO ○ VOICEMAIL ○ NO ANSWER
CONTACT MADE BY:	TIME:
INCIDENT HANDLED BY:	
TREATMENT GIVEN BY:	
FORM COMPLETED BY:	
POSITION:	DATE:
APPROVED BY:	
POSITION:	DATE:

CHILDMINDING ACCIDENT/ INCIDENT REPORT

INCIDENT NO:	INCIDENT DATE:	INCIDENT TIME:
LOCATION:	REPORTED TIME:	REPORTED DATE:

| PERSON INJURED / INVOLVED | ○ STUDENT ○ ACADEMIC STAFF ○ NON-ACADEMIC STAFF
 ○ VISITOR ○ OTHER : |||

FULLNAME:		CLASS:
ADDRESS:		

| NATURE & EXTENT OF INJURIES | ○ GRAZE ○ BUMP ○ CUT ○ FALL ○ NOSEBLEED
 ○ SCRATCHES ○ OTHER: ||||

DETAILS OF INCIDENT / ACCIDENT

| WHAT ACTION WAS TAKEN ? | ○ FIRST AID ○ AMBULLANCE CALLED ○ HOSPITAL ○ POLICE
 ○ OTHER: ||||

WITNESS (ES)	ACTION (S) WHICH COULD HAVE PREVENTED THE INCIDENT
1.	
2.	
3.	

EMERGENCY CONTACT (PARENT / GUARDIAN INFORMATION)

FULLNAME:		
E-MAIL ADDRESS:		PHONE No:
OUTCOME	○ PARENT SPOKEN TO ○ VOICEMAIL	○ NO ANSWER
CONTACT MADE BY:		TIME:
INCIDENT HANDLED BY:		
TREATMENT GIVEN BY:		
FORM COMPLETED BY:		
POSITION:		DATE:
APPROVED BY:		
POSITION:		DATE:

CHILDMINDING ACCIDENT/ INCIDENT REPORT

INCIDENT NO:	INCIDENT DATE:	INCIDENT TIME:
LOCATION:	REPORTED TIME:	REPORTED DATE:

PERSON INJURED / INVOLVED	O STUDENT O ACADEMIC STAFF O NON-ACADEMIC STAFF O VISITOR O OTHER :

FULLNAME:	CLASS:

ADDRESS:

NATURE & EXTENT OF INJURIES	O GRAZE O BUMP O CUT O FALL O NOSEBLEED O SCRATCHES O OTHER:

DETAILS OF INCIDENT / ACCIDENT

WHAT ACTION WAS TAKEN ?	O FIRST AID O AMBULLANCE CALLED O HOSPITAL O POLICE O OTHER:

WITNESS (ES)	ACTION (S) WHICH COULD HAVE PREVENTED THE INCIDENT
1.	
2.	
3.	

EMERGENCY CONTACT (PARENT / GUARDIAN INFORMATION)

FULLNAME:	
E-MAIL ADDRESS:	PHONE No:
OUTCOME	O PARENT SPOKEN TO O VOICEMAIL O NO ANSWER
CONTACT MADE BY:	TIME:
INCIDENT HANDLED BY:	
TREATMENT GIVEN BY:	
FORM COMPLETED BY:	
POSITION:	DATE:
APPROVED BY:	
POSITION:	DATE:

CHILDMINDING ACCIDENT/ INCIDENT REPORT

INCIDENT NO:	INCIDENT DATE:	INCIDENT TIME:
LOCATION:	REPORTED TIME:	REPORTED DATE:

PERSON INJURED / INVOLVED	○ STUDENT ○ ACADEMIC STAFF ○ NON-ACADEMIC STAFF ○ VISITOR ○ OTHER :

FULLNAME:	CLASS:

ADDRESS:	

NATURE & EXTENT OF INJURIES	○ GRAZE ○ BUMP ○ CUT ○ FALL ○ NOSEBLEED ○ SCRATCHES ○ OTHER:

DETAILS OF INCIDENT / ACCIDENT

WHAT ACTION WAS TAKEN ?	○ FIRST AID ○ AMBULLANCE CALLED ○ HOSPITAL ○ POLICE ○ OTHER:

WITNESS (ES)	ACTION (S) WHICH COULD HAVE PREVENTED THE INCIDENT
1.	
2.	
3.	

EMERGENCY CONTACT (PARENT / GUARDIAN INFORMATION)

FULLNAME:		
E-MAIL ADDRESS:	PHONE No:	
OUTCOME	○ PARENT SPOKEN TO ○ VOICEMAIL ○ NO ANSWER	
CONTACT MADE BY:	TIME:	
INCIDENT HANDLED BY:		
TREATMENT GIVEN BY:		
FORM COMPLETED BY:		
POSITION:	DATE:	
APPROVED BY:		
POSITION:	DATE:	

CHILDMINDING ACCIDENT/ INCIDENT REPORT

INCIDENT NO:	INCIDENT DATE:	INCIDENT TIME:
LOCATION:	REPORTED TIME:	REPORTED DATE:

PERSON INJURED / INVOLVED	○ STUDENT ○ ACADEMIC STAFF ○ NON-ACADEMIC STAFF ○ VISITOR ○ OTHER :	

FULLNAME:		CLASS:
ADDRESS:		

NATURE & EXTENT OF INJURIES	○ GRAZE ○ BUMP ○ CUT ○ FALL ○ NOSEBLEED ○ SCRATCHES ○ OTHER:

DETAILS OF INCIDENT / ACCIDENT

WHAT ACTION WAS TAKEN ?	○ FIRST AID ○ AMBULLANCE CALLED ○ HOSPITAL ○ POLICE ○ OTHER:

WITNESS (ES)	ACTION (S) WHICH COULD HAVE PREVENTED THE INCIDENT
1.	
2.	
3.	

EMERGENCY CONTACT (PARENT / GUARDIAN INFORMATION)

FULLNAME:		
E-MAIL ADDRESS:		PHONE No:
OUTCOME	○ PARENT SPOKEN TO ○ VOICEMAIL ○ NO ANSWER	
CONTACT MADE BY:		TIME:
INCIDENT HANDLED BY:		
TREATMENT GIVEN BY:		
FORM COMPLETED BY:		
POSITION:		DATE:
APPROVED BY:		
POSITION:		DATE:

CHILDMINDING ACCIDENT/ INCIDENT REPORT

INCIDENT NO:	INCIDENT DATE:	INCIDENT TIME:
LOCATION:	REPORTED TIME:	REPORTED DATE:

| PERSON INJURED / INVOLVED | O STUDENT   O ACADEMIC STAFF   O NON-ACADEMIC STAFF
O VISITOR   O OTHER : | |

FULLNAME:		CLASS:

ADDRESS:		

| NATURE & EXTENT OF INJURIES | O GRAZE   O BUMP   O CUT   O FALL   O NOSEBLEED
O SCRATCHES   O OTHER: | | | | |

DETAILS OF INCIDENT / ACCIDENT

WHAT ACTION WAS TAKEN ?	O FIRST AID O AMBULLANCE CALLED O HOSPITAL O POLICE O OTHER:

WITNESS (ES)	ACTION (S) WHICH COULD HAVE PREVENTED THE INCIDENT
1.	
2.	
3.	

EMERGENCY CONTACT (PARENT / GUARDIAN INFORMATION)

FULLNAME:		
E-MAIL ADDRESS:		PHONE No:
OUTCOME	O PARENT SPOKEN TO O VOICEMAIL O NO ANSWER	
CONTACT MADE BY:		TIME:
INCIDENT HANDLED BY:		
TREATMENT GIVEN BY:		
FORM COMPLETED BY:		
POSITION:		DATE:
APPROVED BY:		
POSITION:		DATE:

CHILDMINDING ACCIDENT/ INCIDENT REPORT

INCIDENT NO:	INCIDENT DATE:	INCIDENT TIME:
LOCATION:	REPORTED TIME:	REPORTED DATE:

PERSON INJURED / INVOLVED	O STUDENT O ACADEMIC STAFF O NON-ACADEMIC STAFF O VISITOR O OTHER :	

FULLNAME:		CLASS:
ADDRESS:		

NATURE & EXTENT OF INJURIES	O GRAZE O BUMP O CUT O FALL O NOSEBLEED O SCRATCHES O OTHER:

DETAILS OF INCIDENT / ACCIDENT

WHAT ACTION WAS TAKEN ?	O FIRST AID O AMBULLANCE CALLED O HOSPITAL O POLICE O OTHER:

WITNESS (ES)	ACTION (S) WHICH COULD HAVE PREVENTED THE INCIDENT
1.	
2.	
3.	

EMERGENCY CONTACT (PARENT / GUARDIAN INFORMATION)

FULLNAME:		
E-MAIL ADDRESS:		PHONE No:
OUTCOME	O PARENT SPOKEN TO O VOICEMAIL	O NO ANSWER
CONTACT MADE BY:		TIME:
INCIDENT HANDLED BY:		
TREATMENT GIVEN BY:		
FORM COMPLETED BY:		
POSITION:		DATE:
APPROVED BY:		
POSITION:		DATE:

CHILDMINDING ACCIDENT/ INCIDENT REPORT

INCIDENT NO:	INCIDENT DATE:	INCIDENT TIME:
LOCATION:	REPORTED TIME:	REPORTED DATE:

| PERSON INJURED / INVOLVED | ○ STUDENT ○ ACADEMIC STAFF ○ NON-ACADEMIC STAFF
 ○ VISITOR ○ OTHER : | | |

FULLNAME:		CLASS:

ADDRESS:		

NATURE & EXTENT OF INJURIES	○ GRAZE ○ BUMP ○ CUT ○ FALL ○ NOSEBLEED ○ SCRATCHES ○ OTHER:

DETAILS OF INCIDENT / ACCIDENT

_____

_____

_____

_____

WHAT ACTION WAS TAKEN ?	○ FIRST AID ○ AMBULLANCE CALLED ○ HOSPITAL ○ POLICE ○ OTHER:

WITNESS (ES)	ACTION (S) WHICH COULD HAVE PREVENTED THE INCIDENT
1.	
2.	
3.	

EMERGENCY CONTACT (PARENT / GUARDIAN INFORMATION)

FULLNAME:		
E-MAIL ADDRESS:		PHONE No:
OUTCOME	○ PARENT SPOKEN TO ○ VOICEMAIL ○ NO ANSWER	
CONTACT MADE BY:		TIME:
INCIDENT HANDLED BY:		
TREATMENT GIVEN BY:		
FORM COMPLETED BY:		
POSITION:		DATE:
APPROVED BY:		
POSITION:		DATE:

CHILDMINDING ACCIDENT/ INCIDENT REPORT

INCIDENT NO:	INCIDENT DATE:	INCIDENT TIME:
LOCATION:	REPORTED TIME:	REPORTED DATE:

| PERSON INJURED / INVOLVED | O STUDENT   O ACADEMIC STAFF   O NON-ACADEMIC STAFF
O VISITOR   O OTHER : |||

FULLNAME:		CLASS:

ADDRESS:		

| NATURE & EXTENT OF INJURIES | O GRAZE   O BUMP   O CUT   O FALL   O NOSEBLEED
O SCRATCHES   O OTHER: |||

DETAILS OF INCIDENT / ACCIDENT

| WHAT ACTION WAS TAKEN ? | O FIRST AID   O AMBULLANCE CALLED   O HOSPITAL   O POLICE
O OTHER: |||

WITNESS (ES)	ACTION (S) WHICH COULD HAVE PREVENTED THE INCIDENT
1.	
2.	
3.	

EMERGENCY CONTACT (PARENT / GUARDIAN INFORMATION)

FULLNAME:		
E-MAIL ADDRESS:		PHONE No:
OUTCOME	O PARENT SPOKEN TO O VOICEMAIL O NO ANSWER	
CONTACT MADE BY:		TIME:
INCIDENT HANDLED BY:		
TREATMENT GIVEN BY:		
FORM COMPLETED BY:		
POSITION:		DATE:
APPROVED BY:		
POSITION:		DATE:

CHILDMINDING ACCIDENT/ INCIDENT REPORT

INCIDENT NO:	INCIDENT DATE:	INCIDENT TIME:
LOCATION:	REPORTED TIME:	REPORTED DATE:

PERSON INJURED / INVOLVED	O STUDENT O ACADEMIC STAFF O NON-ACADEMIC STAFF O VISITOR O OTHER :

FULLNAME:		CLASS:

ADDRESS:		

NATURE & EXTENT OF INJURIES	O GRAZE O BUMP O CUT O FALL O NOSEBLEED O SCRATCHES O OTHER:

DETAILS OF INCIDENT / ACCIDENT

WHAT ACTION WAS TAKEN ?	O FIRST AID O AMBULLANCE CALLED O HOSPITAL O POLICE O OTHER:

WITNESS (ES)	ACTION (S) WHICH COULD HAVE PREVENTED THE INCIDENT
1.	
2.	
3.	

EMERGENCY CONTACT (PARENT / GUARDIAN INFORMATION)

FULLNAME:		
E-MAIL ADDRESS:		PHONE No:
OUTCOME	O PARENT SPOKEN TO O VOICEMAIL O NO ANSWER	
CONTACT MADE BY:		TIME:
INCIDENT HANDLED BY:		
TREATMENT GIVEN BY:		
FORM COMPLETED BY:		
POSITION:		DATE:
APPROVED BY:		
POSITION:		DATE:

CHILDMINDING ACCIDENT/ INCIDENT REPORT

INCIDENT NO:	INCIDENT DATE:	INCIDENT TIME:
LOCATION:	REPORTED TIME:	REPORTED DATE:

PERSON INJURED / INVOLVED	O STUDENT O ACADEMIC STAFF O NON-ACADEMIC STAFF O VISITOR O OTHER :	

FULLNAME:	CLASS:

ADDRESS:	

NATURE & EXTENT OF INJURIES	O GRAZE O BUMP O CUT O FALL O NOSEBLEED O SCRATCHES O OTHER:

DETAILS OF INCIDENT / ACCIDENT

WHAT ACTION WAS TAKEN ?	O FIRST AID O AMBULLANCE CALLED O HOSPITAL O POLICE O OTHER:

WITNESS (ES)	ACTION (S) WHICH COULD HAVE PREVENTED THE INCIDENT
1.	
2.	
3.	

EMERGENCY CONTACT (PARENT / GUARDIAN INFORMATION)

FULLNAME:	
E-MAIL ADDRESS:	PHONE No:
OUTCOME	O PARENT SPOKEN TO O VOICEMAIL O NO ANSWER
CONTACT MADE BY:	TIME:
INCIDENT HANDLED BY:	
TREATMENT GIVEN BY:	
FORM COMPLETED BY:	
POSITION:	DATE:
APPROVED BY:	
POSITION:	DATE:

CHILDMINDING ACCIDENT/ INCIDENT REPORT

INCIDENT NO:	INCIDENT DATE:	INCIDENT TIME:
LOCATION:	REPORTED TIME:	REPORTED DATE:

| PERSON INJURED / INVOLVED | O STUDENT   O ACADEMIC STAFF   O NON-ACADEMIC STAFF
O VISITOR   O OTHER : | |

FULLNAME:		CLASS:

ADDRESS:

NATURE & EXTENT OF INJURIES	O GRAZE O BUMP O CUT O FALL O NOSEBLEED O SCRATCHES O OTHER:

DETAILS OF INCIDENT / ACCIDENT

WHAT ACTION WAS TAKEN ?	O FIRST AID O AMBULLANCE CALLED O HOSPITAL O POLICE O OTHER:

WITNESS (ES)	ACTION (S) WHICH COULD HAVE PREVENTED THE INCIDENT
1.	
2.	
3.	

EMERGENCY CONTACT (PARENT / GUARDIAN INFORMATION)

FULLNAME:		
E-MAIL ADDRESS:		PHONE No:
OUTCOME	O PARENT SPOKEN TO O VOICEMAIL	O NO ANSWER
CONTACT MADE BY:		TIME:
INCIDENT HANDLED BY:		
TREATMENT GIVEN BY:		
FORM COMPLETED BY:		
POSITION:		DATE:
APPROVED BY:		
POSITION:		DATE:

CHILDMINDING ACCIDENT/ INCIDENT REPORT

INCIDENT NO:	INCIDENT DATE:	INCIDENT TIME:
LOCATION:	REPORTED TIME:	REPORTED DATE:

| PERSON INJURED / INVOLVED | ○ STUDENT   ○ ACADEMIC STAFF   ○ NON-ACADEMIC STAFF
 ○ VISITOR   ○ OTHER : | | |

FULLNAME:		CLASS:

ADDRESS:

NATURE & EXTENT OF INJURIES	○ GRAZE ○ BUMP ○ CUT ○ FALL ○ NOSEBLEED ○ SCRATCHES ○ OTHER:

DETAILS OF INCIDENT / ACCIDENT

WHAT ACTION WAS TAKEN ?	○ FIRST AID ○ AMBULLANCE CALLED ○ HOSPITAL ○ POLICE ○ OTHER:

WITNESS (ES)	ACTION (S) WHICH COULD HAVE PREVENTED THE INCIDENT
1.	
2.	
3.	

EMERGENCY CONTACT (PARENT / GUARDIAN INFORMATION)

FULLNAME:		
E-MAIL ADDRESS:		PHONE No:
OUTCOME	○ PARENT SPOKEN TO ○ VOICEMAIL ○ NO ANSWER	
CONTACT MADE BY:		TIME:
INCIDENT HANDLED BY:		
TREATMENT GIVEN BY:		
FORM COMPLETED BY:		
POSITION:		DATE:
APPROVED BY:		
POSITION:		DATE:

CHILDMINDING ACCIDENT/ INCIDENT REPORT

INCIDENT NO:	INCIDENT DATE:	INCIDENT TIME:
LOCATION:	REPORTED TIME:	REPORTED DATE:

PERSON INJURED / INVOLVED	○ STUDENT ○ ACADEMIC STAFF ○ NON-ACADEMIC STAFF ○ VISITOR ○ OTHER :

FULLNAME:	CLASS:

ADDRESS:

NATURE & EXTENT OF INJURIES	○ GRAZE ○ BUMP ○ CUT ○ FALL ○ NOSEBLEED ○ SCRATCHES ○ OTHER:

DETAILS OF INCIDENT / ACCIDENT

WHAT ACTION WAS TAKEN ?	○ FIRST AID ○ AMBULLANCE CALLED ○ HOSPITAL ○ POLICE ○ OTHER:

WITNESS (ES)	ACTION (S) WHICH COULD HAVE PREVENTED THE INCIDENT
1.	
2.	
3.	

EMERGENCY CONTACT (PARENT / GUARDIAN INFORMATION)

FULLNAME:		
E-MAIL ADDRESS:	PHONE No:	
OUTCOME	○ PARENT SPOKEN TO ○ VOICEMAIL ○ NO ANSWER	
CONTACT MADE BY:	TIME:	
INCIDENT HANDLED BY:		
TREATMENT GIVEN BY:		
FORM COMPLETED BY:		
POSITION:	DATE:	
APPROVED BY:		
POSITION:	DATE:	

CHILDMINDING ACCIDENT/ INCIDENT REPORT

INCIDENT NO:	INCIDENT DATE:	INCIDENT TIME:
LOCATION:	REPORTED TIME:	REPORTED DATE:

PERSON INJURED / INVOLVED	○ STUDENT ○ ACADEMIC STAFF ○ NON-ACADEMIC STAFF ○ VISITOR ○ OTHER :

FULLNAME:	CLASS:

ADDRESS:	

NATURE & EXTENT OF INJURIES	○ GRAZE ○ BUMP ○ CUT ○ FALL ○ NOSEBLEED ○ SCRATCHES ○ OTHER:

DETAILS OF INCIDENT / ACCIDENT

WHAT ACTION WAS TAKEN ?	○ FIRST AID ○ AMBULLANCE CALLED ○ HOSPITAL ○ POLICE ○ OTHER:

WITNESS (ES)	ACTION (S) WHICH COULD HAVE PREVENTED THE INCIDENT
1.	
2.	
3.	

EMERGENCY CONTACT (PARENT / GUARDIAN INFORMATION)

FULLNAME:		
E-MAIL ADDRESS:	PHONE No:	
OUTCOME	○ PARENT SPOKEN TO ○ VOICEMAIL ○ NO ANSWER	
CONTACT MADE BY:	TIME:	
INCIDENT HANDLED BY:		
TREATMENT GIVEN BY:		
FORM COMPLETED BY:		
POSITION:	DATE:	
APPROVED BY:		
POSITION:	DATE:	

CHILDMINDING ACCIDENT/ INCIDENT REPORT

INCIDENT NO:	INCIDENT DATE:	INCIDENT TIME:
LOCATION:	REPORTED TIME:	REPORTED DATE:

PERSON INJURED / INVOLVED	○ STUDENT ○ ACADEMIC STAFF ○ NON-ACADEMIC STAFF ○ VISITOR ○ OTHER :

FULLNAME:	CLASS:

ADDRESS:

NATURE & EXTENT OF INJURIES	○ GRAZE ○ BUMP ○ CUT ○ FALL ○ NOSEBLEED ○ SCRATCHES ○ OTHER:

DETAILS OF INCIDENT / ACCIDENT

WHAT ACTION WAS TAKEN ?	○ FIRST AID ○ AMBULLANCE CALLED ○ HOSPITAL ○ POLICE ○ OTHER:

WITNESS (ES)	ACTION (S) WHICH COULD HAVE PREVENTED THE INCIDENT
1.	
2.	
3.	

EMERGENCY CONTACT (PARENT / GUARDIAN INFORMATION)

FULLNAME:	
E-MAIL ADDRESS:	PHONE No:
OUTCOME	○ PARENT SPOKEN TO ○ VOICEMAIL ○ NO ANSWER
CONTACT MADE BY:	TIME:
INCIDENT HANDLED BY:	
TREATMENT GIVEN BY:	
FORM COMPLETED BY:	
POSITION:	DATE:
APPROVED BY:	
POSITION:	DATE:

CHILDMINDING ACCIDENT/ INCIDENT REPORT

INCIDENT NO:	INCIDENT DATE:		INCIDENT TIME:	
LOCATION:	REPORTED TIME:		REPORTED DATE:	
PERSON INJURED / INVOLVED	○ STUDENT ○ ACADEMIC STAFF ○ NON-ACADEMIC STAFF ○ VISITOR ○ OTHER :			
FULLNAME:			CLASS:	
ADDRESS:				
NATURE & EXTENT OF INJURIES	○ GRAZE ○ BUMP ○ CUT ○ FALL ○ NOSEBLEED ○ SCRATCHES ○ OTHER:			

DETAILS OF INCIDENT / ACCIDENT

WHAT ACTION WAS TAKEN ?	○ FIRST AID ○ AMBULLANCE CALLED ○ HOSPITAL ○ POLICE ○ OTHER:

WITNESS (ES)	ACTION (S) WHICH COULD HAVE PREVENTED THE INCIDENT
1.	
2.	
3.	

EMERGENCY CONTACT (PARENT / GUARDIAN INFORMATION)

FULLNAME:			
E-MAIL ADDRESS:		PHONE No:	
OUTCOME	○ PARENT SPOKEN TO	○ VOICEMAIL	○ NO ANSWER
CONTACT MADE BY:		TIME:	
INCIDENT HANDLED BY:			
TREATMENT GIVEN BY:			
FORM COMPLETED BY:			
POSITION:		DATE:	
APPROVED BY:			
POSITION:		DATE:	

CHILDMINDING ACCIDENT/ INCIDENT REPORT

INCIDENT NO:	INCIDENT DATE:	INCIDENT TIME:
LOCATION:	REPORTED TIME:	REPORTED DATE:

| PERSON INJURED / INVOLVED | O STUDENT   O ACADEMIC STAFF   O NON-ACADEMIC STAFF
 O VISITOR   O OTHER : | |

FULLNAME:		CLASS:

ADDRESS:	

| NATURE & EXTENT OF INJURIES | O GRAZE   O BUMP   O CUT   O FALL   O NOSEBLEED
 O SCRATCHES   O OTHER: |

DETAILS OF INCIDENT / ACCIDENT

| WHAT ACTION WAS TAKEN ? | O FIRST AID   O AMBULLANCE CALLED   O HOSPITAL   O POLICE
 O OTHER: |

WITNESS (ES)	ACTION (S) WHICH COULD HAVE PREVENTED THE INCIDENT
1.	
2.	
3.	

EMERGENCY CONTACT (PARENT / GUARDIAN INFORMATION)

FULLNAME:	

E-MAIL ADDRESS:	PHONE No:

OUTCOME	O PARENT SPOKEN TO O VOICEMAIL O NO ANSWER

CONTACT MADE BY:	TIME:

INCIDENT HANDLED BY:	
TREATMENT GIVEN BY:	
FORM COMPLETED BY:	

POSITION:	DATE:

APPROVED BY:	

POSITION:	DATE:

CHILDMINDING ACCIDENT/ INCIDENT REPORT

INCIDENT NO:	INCIDENT DATE:	INCIDENT TIME:
LOCATION:	REPORTED TIME:	REPORTED DATE:

| PERSON INJURED / INVOLVED | ○ STUDENT ○ ACADEMIC STAFF ○ NON-ACADEMIC STAFF ○ VISITOR ○ OTHER : | | |

FULLNAME:		CLASS:

ADDRESS:

NATURE & EXTENT OF INJURIES	○ GRAZE ○ BUMP ○ CUT ○ FALL ○ NOSEBLEED ○ SCRATCHES ○ OTHER:

DETAILS OF INCIDENT / ACCIDENT

WHAT ACTION WAS TAKEN ?	○ FIRST AID ○ AMBULLANCE CALLED ○ HOSPITAL ○ POLICE ○ OTHER:

WITNESS (ES)	ACTION (S) WHICH COULD HAVE PREVENTED THE INCIDENT
1.	
2.	
3.	

EMERGENCY CONTACT (PARENT / GUARDIAN INFORMATION)

FULLNAME:		
E-MAIL ADDRESS:		PHONE No:
OUTCOME	○ PARENT SPOKEN TO ○ VOICEMAIL ○ NO ANSWER	
CONTACT MADE BY:		TIME:
INCIDENT HANDLED BY:		
TREATMENT GIVEN BY:		
FORM COMPLETED BY:		
POSITION:		DATE:
APPROVED BY:		
POSITION:		DATE:

CHILDMINDING ACCIDENT/ INCIDENT REPORT

INCIDENT NO:	INCIDENT DATE:	INCIDENT TIME:
LOCATION:	REPORTED TIME:	REPORTED DATE:

| PERSON INJURED / INVOLVED | O STUDENT O ACADEMIC STAFF O NON-ACADEMIC STAFF O VISITOR O OTHER : | | |

FULLNAME:		CLASS:

ADDRESS:		

NATURE & EXTENT OF INJURIES	O GRAZE O BUMP O CUT O FALL O NOSEBLEED O SCRATCHES O OTHER:

DETAILS OF INCIDENT / ACCIDENT

WHAT ACTION WAS TAKEN ?	O FIRST AID O AMBULLANCE CALLED O HOSPITAL O POLICE O OTHER:

WITNESS (ES)	ACTION (S) WHICH COULD HAVE PREVENTED THE INCIDENT
1.	
2.	
3.	

EMERGENCY CONTACT (PARENT / GUARDIAN INFORMATION)

FULLNAME:		
E-MAIL ADDRESS:		PHONE No:
OUTCOME	O PARENT SPOKEN TO O VOICEMAIL O NO ANSWER	
CONTACT MADE BY:		TIME:
INCIDENT HANDLED BY:		
TREATMENT GIVEN BY:		
FORM COMPLETED BY:		
POSITION:		DATE:
APPROVED BY:		
POSITION:		DATE:

CHILDMINDING ACCIDENT/ INCIDENT REPORT

INCIDENT NO:	INCIDENT DATE:	INCIDENT TIME:
LOCATION:	REPORTED TIME:	REPORTED DATE:

PERSON INJURED / INVOLVED	○ STUDENT ○ ACADEMIC STAFF ○ NON-ACADEMIC STAFF ○ VISITOR ○ OTHER :	

FULLNAME:	CLASS:

ADDRESS:	

NATURE & EXTENT OF INJURIES	○ GRAZE ○ BUMP ○ CUT ○ FALL ○ NOSEBLEED ○ SCRATCHES ○ OTHER:

DETAILS OF INCIDENT / ACCIDENT

WHAT ACTION WAS TAKEN ?	○ FIRST AID ○ AMBULLANCE CALLED ○ HOSPITAL ○ POLICE ○ OTHER:

WITNESS (ES)	ACTION (S) WHICH COULD HAVE PREVENTED THE INCIDENT
1.	
2.	
3.	

EMERGENCY CONTACT (PARENT / GUARDIAN INFORMATION)

FULLNAME:		
E-MAIL ADDRESS:		PHONE No:
OUTCOME	○ PARENT SPOKEN TO ○ VOICEMAIL	○ NO ANSWER
CONTACT MADE BY:		TIME:
INCIDENT HANDLED BY:		
TREATMENT GIVEN BY:		
FORM COMPLETED BY:		
POSITION:		DATE:
APPROVED BY:		
POSITION:		DATE:

CHILDMINDING ACCIDENT/ INCIDENT REPORT

INCIDENT NO:	INCIDENT DATE:	INCIDENT TIME:
LOCATION:	REPORTED TIME:	REPORTED DATE:

PERSON INJURED / INVOLVED	O STUDENT O ACADEMIC STAFF O NON-ACADEMIC STAFF O VISITOR O OTHER :	

FULLNAME:	CLASS:

ADDRESS:	

NATURE & EXTENT OF INJURIES	O GRAZE O BUMP O CUT O FALL O NOSEBLEED O SCRATCHES O OTHER:

DETAILS OF INCIDENT / ACCIDENT

WHAT ACTION WAS TAKEN ?	O FIRST AID O AMBULLANCE CALLED O HOSPITAL O POLICE O OTHER:

WITNESS (ES)	ACTION (S) WHICH COULD HAVE PREVENTED THE INCIDENT
1.	
2.	
3.	

EMERGENCY CONTACT (PARENT / GUARDIAN INFORMATION)

FULLNAME:	
E-MAIL ADDRESS:	PHONE No:
OUTCOME	O PARENT SPOKEN TO O VOICEMAIL O NO ANSWER
CONTACT MADE BY:	TIME:
INCIDENT HANDLED BY:	
TREATMENT GIVEN BY:	
FORM COMPLETED BY:	
POSITION:	DATE:
APPROVED BY:	
POSITION:	DATE:

CHILDMINDING ACCIDENT/ INCIDENT REPORT

INCIDENT NO:	INCIDENT DATE:	INCIDENT TIME:
LOCATION:	REPORTED TIME:	REPORTED DATE:

| PERSON INJURED / INVOLVED | O STUDENT   O ACADEMIC STAFF   O NON-ACADEMIC STAFF
 O VISITOR   O OTHER : | | |

FULLNAME:	CLASS:

ADDRESS:

NATURE & EXTENT OF INJURIES	O GRAZE O BUMP O CUT O FALL O NOSEBLEED O SCRATCHES O OTHER:

DETAILS OF INCIDENT / ACCIDENT

WHAT ACTION WAS TAKEN ?	O FIRST AID O AMBULLANCE CALLED O HOSPITAL O POLICE O OTHER:

WITNESS (ES)	ACTION (S) WHICH COULD HAVE PREVENTED THE INCIDENT
1.	
2.	
3.	

EMERGENCY CONTACT (PARENT / GUARDIAN INFORMATION)

FULLNAME:		
E-MAIL ADDRESS:	PHONE No:	
OUTCOME	O PARENT SPOKEN TO O VOICEMAIL O NO ANSWER	
CONTACT MADE BY:	TIME:	
INCIDENT HANDLED BY:		
TREATMENT GIVEN BY:		
FORM COMPLETED BY:		
POSITION:	DATE:	
APPROVED BY:		
POSITION:	DATE:	

CHILDMINDING ACCIDENT/ INCIDENT REPORT

INCIDENT NO:	INCIDENT DATE:	INCIDENT TIME:
LOCATION:	REPORTED TIME:	REPORTED DATE:

PERSON INJURED / INVOLVED	⊙ STUDENT ⊙ ACADEMIC STAFF ⊙ NON-ACADEMIC STAFF ⊙ VISITOR ⊙ OTHER :

FULLNAME:	CLASS:

ADDRESS:	

NATURE & EXTENT OF INJURIES	⊙ GRAZE ⊙ BUMP ⊙ CUT ⊙ FALL ⊙ NOSEBLEED ⊙ SCRATCHES ⊙ OTHER:

DETAILS OF INCIDENT / ACCIDENT

WHAT ACTION WAS TAKEN ?	⊙ FIRST AID ⊙ AMBULLANCE CALLED ⊙ HOSPITAL ⊙ POLICE ⊙ OTHER:

WITNESS (ES)	ACTION (S) WHICH COULD HAVE PREVENTED THE INCIDENT
1.	
2.	
3.	

EMERGENCY CONTACT (PARENT / GUARDIAN INFORMATION)

FULLNAME:		
E-MAIL ADDRESS:	PHONE No:	
OUTCOME	⊙ PARENT SPOKEN TO ⊙ VOICEMAIL ⊙ NO ANSWER	
CONTACT MADE BY:	TIME:	
INCIDENT HANDLED BY:		
TREATMENT GIVEN BY:		
FORM COMPLETED BY:		
POSITION:	DATE:	
APPROVED BY:		
POSITION:	DATE:	

CHILDMINDING ACCIDENT/ INCIDENT REPORT

INCIDENT NO:	INCIDENT DATE:		INCIDENT TIME:
LOCATION:	REPORTED TIME:		REPORTED DATE:
PERSON INJURED / INVOLVED	○ STUDENT ○ ACADEMIC STAFF ○ NON-ACADEMIC STAFF ○ VISITOR ○ OTHER :		
FULLNAME:		CLASS:	
ADDRESS:			
NATURE & EXTENT OF INJURIES	○ GRAZE ○ BUMP ○ CUT ○ FALL ○ NOSEBLEED ○ SCRATCHES ○ OTHER:		

DETAILS OF INCIDENT / ACCIDENT

WHAT ACTION WAS TAKEN ?	○ FIRST AID ○ AMBULLANCE CALLED ○ HOSPITAL ○ POLICE ○ OTHER:

WITNESS (ES)	ACTION (S) WHICH COULD HAVE PREVENTED THE INCIDENT
1.	
2.	
3.	

EMERGENCY CONTACT (PARENT / GUARDIAN INFORMATION)

FULLNAME:			
E-MAIL ADDRESS:		PHONE No:	
OUTCOME	○ PARENT SPOKEN TO	○ VOICEMAIL	○ NO ANSWER
CONTACT MADE BY:		TIME:	
INCIDENT HANDLED BY:			
TREATMENT GIVEN BY:			
FORM COMPLETED BY:			
POSITION:		DATE:	
APPROVED BY:			
POSITION:		DATE:	

CHILDMINDING ACCIDENT/ INCIDENT REPORT

INCIDENT NO:	INCIDENT DATE:	INCIDENT TIME:
LOCATION:	REPORTED TIME:	REPORTED DATE:

| PERSON INJURED / INVOLVED | ○ STUDENT   ○ ACADEMIC STAFF   ○ NON-ACADEMIC STAFF ○ VISITOR   ○ OTHER : |

FULLNAME:		CLASS:
ADDRESS:		

| NATURE & EXTENT OF INJURIES | ○ GRAZE   ○ BUMP   ○ CUT   ○ FALL   ○ NOSEBLEED ○ SCRATCHES   ○ OTHER: |

DETAILS OF INCIDENT / ACCIDENT

| WHAT ACTION WAS TAKEN ? | ○ FIRST AID   ○ AMBULLANCE CALLED   ○ HOSPITAL   ○ POLICE ○ OTHER: |

WITNESS (ES)	ACTION (S) WHICH COULD HAVE PREVENTED THE INCIDENT
1.	
2.	
3.	

EMERGENCY CONTACT (PARENT / GUARDIAN INFORMATION)

FULLNAME:		
E-MAIL ADDRESS:		PHONE No:
OUTCOME	○ PARENT SPOKEN TO ○ VOICEMAIL ○ NO ANSWER	
CONTACT MADE BY:		TIME:
INCIDENT HANDLED BY:		
TREATMENT GIVEN BY:		
FORM COMPLETED BY:		
POSITION:		DATE:
APPROVED BY:		
POSITION:		DATE:

CHILDMINDING ACCIDENT/ INCIDENT REPORT

INCIDENT NO:	INCIDENT DATE:	INCIDENT TIME:
LOCATION:	REPORTED TIME:	REPORTED DATE:

PERSON INJURED / INVOLVED	O STUDENT O ACADEMIC STAFF O NON-ACADEMIC STAFF O VISITOR O OTHER :

FULLNAME:	CLASS:

ADDRESS:

NATURE & EXTENT OF INJURIES	O GRAZE O BUMP O CUT O FALL O NOSEBLEED O SCRATCHES O OTHER:

DETAILS OF INCIDENT / ACCIDENT

WHAT ACTION WAS TAKEN ?	O FIRST AID O AMBULLANCE CALLED O HOSPITAL O POLICE O OTHER:

WITNESS (ES)	ACTION (S) WHICH COULD HAVE PREVENTED THE INCIDENT
1.	
2.	
3.	

EMERGENCY CONTACT (PARENT / GUARDIAN INFORMATION)

FULLNAME:	
E-MAIL ADDRESS:	PHONE No:
OUTCOME	O PARENT SPOKEN TO O VOICEMAIL O NO ANSWER
CONTACT MADE BY:	TIME:
INCIDENT HANDLED BY:	
TREATMENT GIVEN BY:	
FORM COMPLETED BY:	
POSITION:	DATE:
APPROVED BY:	
POSITION:	DATE:

CHILDMINDING ACCIDENT/ INCIDENT REPORT

INCIDENT NO:	INCIDENT DATE:	INCIDENT TIME:
LOCATION:	REPORTED TIME:	REPORTED DATE:

PERSON INJURED / INVOLVED	○ STUDENT ○ ACADEMIC STAFF ○ NON-ACADEMIC STAFF ○ VISITOR ○ OTHER :

FULLNAME:		CLASS:
ADDRESS:		

NATURE & EXTENT OF INJURIES	○ GRAZE ○ BUMP ○ CUT ○ FALL ○ NOSEBLEED ○ SCRATCHES ○ OTHER:

DETAILS OF INCIDENT / ACCIDENT

WHAT ACTION WAS TAKEN ?	○ FIRST AID ○ AMBULLANCE CALLED ○ HOSPITAL ○ POLICE ○ OTHER:

WITNESS (ES)	ACTION (S) WHICH COULD HAVE PREVENTED THE INCIDENT
1.	
2.	
3.	

EMERGENCY CONTACT (PARENT / GUARDIAN INFORMATION)

FULLNAME:		
E-MAIL ADDRESS:		PHONE No:
OUTCOME	○ PARENT SPOKEN TO ○ VOICEMAIL	○ NO ANSWER
CONTACT MADE BY:		TIME:
INCIDENT HANDLED BY:		
TREATMENT GIVEN BY:		
FORM COMPLETED BY:		
POSITION:		DATE:
APPROVED BY:		
POSITION:		DATE:

CHILDMINDING ACCIDENT/ INCIDENT REPORT

INCIDENT NO:	INCIDENT DATE:	INCIDENT TIME:
LOCATION:	REPORTED TIME:	REPORTED DATE:

PERSON INJURED / INVOLVED	O STUDENT O ACADEMIC STAFF O NON-ACADEMIC STAFF O VISITOR O OTHER :

FULLNAME:	CLASS:

ADDRESS:	

NATURE & EXTENT OF INJURIES	O GRAZE O BUMP O CUT O FALL O NOSEBLEED O SCRATCHES O OTHER:

DETAILS OF INCIDENT / ACCIDENT

WHAT ACTION WAS TAKEN ?	O FIRST AID O AMBULLANCE CALLED O HOSPITAL O POLICE O OTHER:

WITNESS (ES)	ACTION (S) WHICH COULD HAVE PREVENTED THE INCIDENT
1.	
2.	
3.	

EMERGENCY CONTACT (PARENT / GUARDIAN INFORMATION)

FULLNAME:		
E-MAIL ADDRESS:		PHONE No:
OUTCOME	O PARENT SPOKEN TO O VOICEMAIL O NO ANSWER	
CONTACT MADE BY:		TIME:
INCIDENT HANDLED BY:		
TREATMENT GIVEN BY:		
FORM COMPLETED BY:		
POSITION:		DATE:
APPROVED BY:		
POSITION:		DATE:

CHILDMINDING ACCIDENT/ INCIDENT REPORT

INCIDENT NO:	INCIDENT DATE:	INCIDENT TIME:
LOCATION:	REPORTED TIME:	REPORTED DATE:

PERSON INJURED / INVOLVED	O STUDENT O ACADEMIC STAFF O NON-ACADEMIC STAFF O VISITOR O OTHER :		

FULLNAME:		CLASS:

ADDRESS:

NATURE & EXTENT OF INJURIES	O GRAZE O BUMP O CUT O FALL O NOSEBLEED O SCRATCHES O OTHER:

DETAILS OF INCIDENT / ACCIDENT

WHAT ACTION WAS TAKEN ?	O FIRST AID O AMBULLANCE CALLED O HOSPITAL O POLICE O OTHER:

WITNESS (ES)	ACTION (S) WHICH COULD HAVE PREVENTED THE INCIDENT
1.	
2.	
3.	

EMERGENCY CONTACT (PARENT / GUARDIAN INFORMATION)

FULLNAME:		
E-MAIL ADDRESS:		PHONE No:
OUTCOME	O PARENT SPOKEN TO O VOICEMAIL O NO ANSWER	
CONTACT MADE BY:		TIME:
INCIDENT HANDLED BY:		
TREATMENT GIVEN BY:		
FORM COMPLETED BY:		
POSITION:		DATE:
APPROVED BY:		
POSITION:		DATE:

CHILDMINDING ACCIDENT/ INCIDENT REPORT

INCIDENT NO:	INCIDENT DATE:	INCIDENT TIME:
LOCATION:	REPORTED TIME:	REPORTED DATE:

PERSON INJURED / INVOLVED	○ STUDENT ○ ACADEMIC STAFF ○ NON-ACADEMIC STAFF ○ VISITOR ○ OTHER :

FULLNAME:	CLASS:

ADDRESS:

NATURE & EXTENT OF INJURIES	○ GRAZE ○ BUMP ○ CUT ○ FALL ○ NOSEBLEED ○ SCRATCHES ○ OTHER:

DETAILS OF INCIDENT / ACCIDENT

WHAT ACTION WAS TAKEN ?	○ FIRST AID ○ AMBULLANCE CALLED ○ HOSPITAL ○ POLICE ○ OTHER:

WITNESS (ES)	ACTION (S) WHICH COULD HAVE PREVENTED THE INCIDENT
1.	
2.	
3.	

EMERGENCY CONTACT (PARENT / GUARDIAN INFORMATION)

FULLNAME:		
E-MAIL ADDRESS:	PHONE No:	
OUTCOME	○ PARENT SPOKEN TO ○ VOICEMAIL ○ NO ANSWER	
CONTACT MADE BY:	TIME:	
INCIDENT HANDLED BY:		
TREATMENT GIVEN BY:		
FORM COMPLETED BY:		
POSITION:	DATE:	
APPROVED BY:		
POSITION:	DATE:	

CHILDMINDING ACCIDENT/ INCIDENT REPORT

INCIDENT NO:	INCIDENT DATE:	INCIDENT TIME:
LOCATION:	REPORTED TIME:	REPORTED DATE:

| PERSON INJURED / INVOLVED | ○ STUDENT ○ ACADEMIC STAFF ○ NON-ACADEMIC STAFF ○ VISITOR ○ OTHER : | | |

FULLNAME:		CLASS:

ADDRESS:	

NATURE & EXTENT OF INJURIES	○ GRAZE ○ BUMP ○ CUT ○ FALL ○ NOSEBLEED ○ SCRATCHES ○ OTHER:

DETAILS OF INCIDENT / ACCIDENT

WHAT ACTION WAS TAKEN ?	○ FIRST AID ○ AMBULLANCE CALLED ○ HOSPITAL ○ POLICE ○ OTHER:

WITNESS (ES)	ACTION (S) WHICH COULD HAVE PREVENTED THE INCIDENT
1.	
2.	
3.	

EMERGENCY CONTACT (PARENT / GUARDIAN INFORMATION)

FULLNAME:	
E-MAIL ADDRESS:	PHONE No:
OUTCOME	○ PARENT SPOKEN TO ○ VOICEMAIL ○ NO ANSWER
CONTACT MADE BY:	TIME:
INCIDENT HANDLED BY:	
TREATMENT GIVEN BY:	
FORM COMPLETED BY:	
POSITION:	DATE:
APPROVED BY:	
POSITION:	DATE:

CHILDMINDING ACCIDENT/ INCIDENT REPORT

INCIDENT NO:	INCIDENT DATE:	INCIDENT TIME:
LOCATION:	REPORTED TIME:	REPORTED DATE:

| PERSON INJURED / INVOLVED | ○ STUDENT   ○ ACADEMIC STAFF   ○ NON-ACADEMIC STAFF
○ VISITOR   ○ OTHER : |||

FULLNAME:	CLASS:

ADDRESS:	

| NATURE & EXTENT OF INJURIES | ○ GRAZE   ○ BUMP   ○ CUT   ○ FALL   ○ NOSEBLEED
○ SCRATCHES   ○ OTHER: |

DETAILS OF INCIDENT / ACCIDENT

WHAT ACTION WAS TAKEN ?	○ FIRST AID ○ AMBULLANCE CALLED ○ HOSPITAL ○ POLICE ○ OTHER:

WITNESS (ES)	ACTION (S) WHICH COULD HAVE PREVENTED THE INCIDENT
1.	
2.	
3.	

EMERGENCY CONTACT (PARENT / GUARDIAN INFORMATION)

FULLNAME:	
E-MAIL ADDRESS:	PHONE No:
OUTCOME	○ PARENT SPOKEN TO ○ VOICEMAIL ○ NO ANSWER
CONTACT MADE BY:	TIME:
INCIDENT HANDLED BY:	
TREATMENT GIVEN BY:	
FORM COMPLETED BY:	
POSITION:	DATE:
APPROVED BY:	
POSITION:	DATE:

CHILDMINDING ACCIDENT/ INCIDENT REPORT

INCIDENT NO:	INCIDENT DATE:	INCIDENT TIME:
LOCATION:	REPORTED TIME:	REPORTED DATE:

| PERSON INJURED / INVOLVED | ○ STUDENT ○ ACADEMIC STAFF ○ NON-ACADEMIC STAFF
 ○ VISITOR ○ OTHER : |||

FULLNAME:		CLASS:

| ADDRESS: ||||

| NATURE & EXTENT OF INJURIES | ○ GRAZE ○ BUMP ○ CUT ○ FALL ○ NOSEBLEED
 ○ SCRATCHES ○ OTHER: |||||

DETAILS OF INCIDENT / ACCIDENT

| WHAT ACTION WAS TAKEN ? | ○ FIRST AID ○ AMBULLANCE CALLED ○ HOSPITAL ○ POLICE
 ○ OTHER: ||||

WITNESS (ES)	ACTION (S) WHICH COULD HAVE PREVENTED THE INCIDENT
1.	
2.	
3.	

EMERGENCY CONTACT (PARENT / GUARDIAN INFORMATION)

FULLNAME:		
E-MAIL ADDRESS:		PHONE No:
OUTCOME	○ PARENT SPOKEN TO ○ VOICEMAIL ○ NO ANSWER	
CONTACT MADE BY:		TIME:
INCIDENT HANDLED BY:		
TREATMENT GIVEN BY:		
FORM COMPLETED BY:		
POSITION:		DATE:
APPROVED BY:		
POSITION:		DATE:

CHILDMINDING ACCIDENT/ INCIDENT REPORT

INCIDENT NO:	INCIDENT DATE:	INCIDENT TIME:
LOCATION:	REPORTED TIME:	REPORTED DATE:

PERSON INJURED / INVOLVED	O STUDENT O ACADEMIC STAFF O NON-ACADEMIC STAFF O VISITOR O OTHER :

FULLNAME:	CLASS:

ADDRESS:	

NATURE & EXTENT OF INJURIES	O GRAZE O BUMP O CUT O FALL O NOSEBLEED O SCRATCHES O OTHER:

DETAILS OF INCIDENT / ACCIDENT

WHAT ACTION WAS TAKEN ?	O FIRST AID O AMBULLANCE CALLED O HOSPITAL O POLICE O OTHER:

WITNESS (ES)	ACTION (S) WHICH COULD HAVE PREVENTED THE INCIDENT
1.	
2.	
3.	

EMERGENCY CONTACT (PARENT / GUARDIAN INFORMATION)

FULLNAME:	
E-MAIL ADDRESS:	PHONE No:
OUTCOME	O PARENT SPOKEN TO O VOICEMAIL O NO ANSWER
CONTACT MADE BY:	TIME:
INCIDENT HANDLED BY:	
TREATMENT GIVEN BY:	
FORM COMPLETED BY:	
POSITION:	DATE:
APPROVED BY:	
POSITION:	DATE:

CHILDMINDING ACCIDENT/ INCIDENT REPORT

INCIDENT NO:	INCIDENT DATE:	INCIDENT TIME:
LOCATION:	REPORTED TIME:	REPORTED DATE:

| PERSON INJURED / INVOLVED | O STUDENT   O ACADEMIC STAFF   O NON-ACADEMIC STAFF
O VISITOR   O OTHER : | |

FULLNAME:		CLASS:

ADDRESS:

NATURE & EXTENT OF INJURIES	O GRAZE O BUMP O CUT O FALL O NOSEBLEED O SCRATCHES O OTHER:

DETAILS OF INCIDENT / ACCIDENT

WHAT ACTION WAS TAKEN ?	O FIRST AID O AMBULLANCE CALLED O HOSPITAL O POLICE O OTHER:

WITNESS (ES)	ACTION (S) WHICH COULD HAVE PREVENTED THE INCIDENT
1.	
2.	
3.	

EMERGENCY CONTACT (PARENT / GUARDIAN INFORMATION)

FULLNAME:		
E-MAIL ADDRESS:		PHONE No:
OUTCOME	O PARENT SPOKEN TO O VOICEMAIL O NO ANSWER	
CONTACT MADE BY:		TIME:
INCIDENT HANDLED BY:		
TREATMENT GIVEN BY:		
FORM COMPLETED BY:		
POSITION:		DATE:
APPROVED BY:		
POSITION:		DATE:

CHILDMINDING ACCIDENT/ INCIDENT REPORT

INCIDENT NO:	INCIDENT DATE:	INCIDENT TIME:
LOCATION:	REPORTED TIME:	REPORTED DATE:

PERSON INJURED / INVOLVED	○ STUDENT ○ ACADEMIC STAFF ○ NON-ACADEMIC STAFF ○ VISITOR ○ OTHER :	
FULLNAME:		CLASS:
ADDRESS:		
NATURE & EXTENT OF INJURIES	○ GRAZE ○ BUMP ○ CUT ○ FALL ○ NOSEBLEED ○ SCRATCHES ○ OTHER:	

DETAILS OF INCIDENT / ACCIDENT

WHAT ACTION WAS TAKEN ?	○ FIRST AID ○ AMBULLANCE CALLED ○ HOSPITAL ○ POLICE ○ OTHER:

WITNESS (ES)	ACTION (S) WHICH COULD HAVE PREVENTED THE INCIDENT
1.	
2.	
3.	

EMERGENCY CONTACT (PARENT / GUARDIAN INFORMATION)

FULLNAME:		
E-MAIL ADDRESS:		PHONE No:
OUTCOME	○ PARENT SPOKEN TO	○ VOICEMAIL ○ NO ANSWER
CONTACT MADE BY:		TIME:
INCIDENT HANDLED BY:		
TREATMENT GIVEN BY:		
FORM COMPLETED BY:		
POSITION:		DATE:
APPROVED BY:		
POSITION:		DATE:

Thank you!

We hope you enjoyed our book.

As a small family company, your feedback is very important to us .

Please let us know how you like our book at :

pickme.readme@gmail.com